Also by Betty Rohde:

So Fat, Low Fat, No Fat

More
So Fat,
Low Fat,
No Fat

Betty Rohde

A FIRESIDE BOOK Published by Simon & Schuster

New York   London   Toronto   Sydney   Tokyo   Singapore

FIRESIDE
Rockefeller Center
1230 Avenue of the Americas
New York, NY 10020

FIRESIDE and colophon are registered trademarks
of Simon & Schuster Inc.

Designed by Bonni Leon-Berman

Manufactured in the United States of America

10   9   8   7   6   5   4   3   2   1

Library of Congress Cataloging-in-Publication Data
Rohde, Betty.
More so fat, low fat, no fat / Betty Rohde.
p.   cm.
Includes index.
1. Low-fat diet—recipes.   I. Title.
RM237.7.R627   1996
641.5'638—dc20   95-42033
CIP

ISBN 0-684-81574-5

Dedication of this book is again to Bob, as he is still my guinea pig, official taster, and critical critiquer, and he is still alive. He certainly has been an asset to each and every one of you, as well as to me. You don't have any idea how many rejects get produced along with the accepted. He is just about to get a little concerned with what is on his plate in the evening. Seems like it doesn't matter—he eats it and does his critiquing and believe me he does express his opinion, for which I am very grateful, even if I don't agree. You know what Billy Graham said about a married couple: "If you both agreed on everything, one of you would be unnecessary." Well, I wouldn't ever want him to think I am unnecessary, so I see to it that I remain necessary.

Thank you, Bob, for being such a caring and concerned companion. Most of all, thank you for your taste buds and for some of your opinions. Lifetime love surrounds you.

MARRIAGE STEW

2 concerned persons
2 cups love
2 pinches understanding
2 teaspoons patience
2 cans trust
2 well-rounded measures of sex
Plenty of honest friendship

Combine the 2 concerned persons and 2 cups of love. Blend with understanding and patience. Beat lightly with a spoonful of laughter. Now add the 2 cans of trust and pour the mixture into the casserole of life. This is also the time to add tears, dreams, touching, and remembering. As the mixture is simmering, sauté sex in tenderness. Cook to taste, garnish with a kiss or two, and serve with honest friendship.

Author unknown

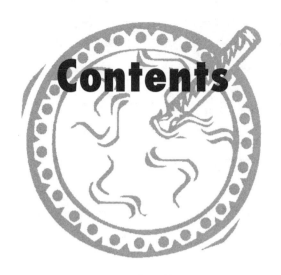

Contents

"THE TWENTY-THIRD DIET"

PROVERBS 17:22 SAYS: "A MERRY HEART DOETH GOOD LIKE A MEDICINE."

My appetite is my shepherd.
I shall always want.
It maketh me to sit down and stuff myself.
It leadeth me to the refrigerator repeatedly.
It destroyeth my shape and my health.
It leadeth me in the paths of fast food, for burgers and fries.
Yea, though I know that I gaineth,
I will not stop eating for the food tasteth so good.
The ice cream and the cookies, they comfort me.
When the table is spread before me, it exciteth me, for I know that soon
I will indulge in food that is good for me and tastes normal.
As I fill my plate continually, my heart and waistline grow stronger and smaller.
For I have found *More So Fat, Low Fat, No Fat*.
Surely bulges and excess weight shall leave me all the days of my life,
And I shall eat good food and live healthier forever.

Amen.

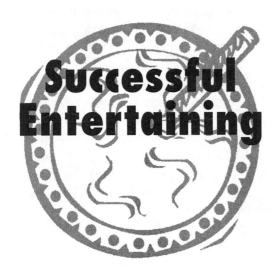

Successful Entertaining

Entertaining can be very rewarding without being taxing on the hostess. The main thing is to use your head. My dad always told me, "Girl, if you don't use your head, you might as well have two rear ends." Now that I am older I must say that I agree with him. One moment to plot a plan will save you many hours of grief.

Decide how many guests you are going to have. Don't overload yourself, or first thing you know you'll have turned a fun affair into a frantic work project.

Decide what type of entertaining—casual, formal, theme, holiday, etc. You can have lots of fun with little effort. We have these friends—there are eight of us—and somehow we got the nickname "the Mangy Gang." We do all kinds of fun things, including theme-type parties. For instance, my friend Jean once had a Road-kill party. She made up menus that had all kinds of entrees like Chunk of Skunk, Snake Steak, Possum Pie, Owl Stew, and Guess This Mess. She wrote one out and copied it on a copy machine, and she and her husband dressed really neat in vests, jeans, chef hats, etc. They stood at each table and took orders as if we were at a restaurant. Of course everyone was getting the same thing (it was a New Year's party and we were having black-eyed peas and so on) but it was really fun ordering. She served on (tin) pie plates, with one spoon to eat with, fruit jars for glasses, weeds in the center of the tables, and so forth. This was a wonderful party, but there was one thing that surprised her, so all the planning in the world won't keep the unexpected from happening. What happened was we all found out the party theme, secretly talked, and every one of us wore something we dug out of the depths of our past to do with fur. I have an old rabbit coat, twenty-five years old. Bob wore overalls, tied a couple of our grandchildren's stuffed toys by the leg with a rope, and threw these over his shoulder like he had picked them up off the road. One of our group wore an old fur hat. You can really have a lot of fun doing simple inexpensive things like this. We all arrived at her house at the same time. You should have seen her face! We do have pictures.

Try your recipes ahead of time. Never advertise your menu in advance. Last-minute disasters can cause many changes that they never need to know about.

Always save time for yourself to get dressed. Look as if you haven't been doing a thing.

When entertaining special guests, like the boss or the husband's boss, don't be afraid of the menu. Don't think just because they are the boss that you have to spend a lot of money or knock yourself out with your menu. I will never forget one time I was taking on a major entertaining project. My first husband's boss was in town for an oil show, along with reps from all over the country. I did my head work—when they all arrived for a sit-down dinner I think that I was most popular. I served in the kitchen and had a regular old-fashioned beans and corn bread, ham, and potatoes dinner. I thought the men were going to kill themselves eating. The boss made the comment, "I get so tired of being served steaks everywhere I go, I am really enjoying this wonderful real food." Steaks are nice, but—everyone likes good, down-home country cooking. Try it! Doesn't have to be beans and corn bread; whatever is your specialty, your environment, your lifestyle, if it be New England lobster or Louisiana crawfish. Just be yourself, be comfortable, be friends, have fun, enjoy life. It is snuffed out too quick and too soon. Smile at everyone you meet. It makes them think you're up to no good, and wonder what's *she* been eating.

Remember Kahlúa and Cool Whip. You can cover up a multitude of sins and mistakes as well as enhance the simplest little effort with the two of these.

You may try a Road Crawl party. This is where you go from one house to another for your dinner. Some call it a Progressive party. We call it Road Crawl. One person has the before-dinner drinks, next house has hors d'oeuvres, next house has soup, next salad, next main course, next dessert. The number of courses depends on the size of the group.

If you are looking for an extraordinary way to entertain without the hassle of the menu and all the decisions, why not try a Tasting Party?

Make out your guest list and ask each person to bring something to do with the theme you are planning, such as a *So Fat, Low Fat, No Fat* party. Have each one make a recipe from their cookbook or provide them with recipes, or just see what each person can come up with in the low-no fat category. You're in for a lot of fun and a healthy party as well.

Keep the party casual—food, dress, decor, buffet-style service all casual. Eat and drink as you please, visit, discuss the recipes, enjoy the food and friends.

Parties can be so much fun and so easy. I feel people don't entertain enough these days. I think we have gotten so formal that we have neglected entertaining because of the dreaded work and worry. Forget it, be comfortable, enjoy your life.

I have also had very successful wine-tasting parties. On the invitation to the wine tasting, add the letters B.Y.O.B. and make sure the guests are told that the last B stands for Not Tried Before Bottle of wine, or their favorite wine. Everyone who comes will bring a different kind of wine. Provide small glasses for a taste of each one, as well as the snacks—fat-free, of course. We have found out about some of the nicest wines this way. In the summer you can also do this with beer if you're planning a patio party or cookout.

Serve food that complements either the wine or beer theme, whichever the case may be.

You may even want to have a judging. Give small pieces of paper and pencils for your guests to make their choice and vote on the "Best of the Bash."

My most fearful nightmare is that on the night of the party, only two people show up, or that my food and drinks run out after the first ten minutes. I don't know which one I fear the most. To avoid these fears, I try to plan ahead with the following steps:

- Guest list: Decide whom you are inviting and write down the names to avoid forgetting someone.
- Invitations: They can be as informal as a phone call or a quick chat with someone in the hall or at church. Just be sure the communication is clear. Poor communication is the root of all evil. Be it a party or a marriage, good communication is the key. The time, place, kind of party—formal, informal, birthday, whatever the occasion—be sure everyone gets all the statistics. Wouldn't you hate to show up in that cute devil suit grinning from ear to ear at the company party instead of the costume party?

  It is also appropriate to limit the time of a cocktail party. The invitation may say "4 to 7" or "Stop by any time between 4 and 8 P.M." for an open house.

- SCHEDULE

  Two to three weeks in advance
  Plan menu and cooking schedule.
  Check nonfood supplies.
  Begin purchase of nonperishables; arrange for rentals.

  One to two weeks in advance
  Begin purchasing beverages.
  Begin preparing foods that can be made in advance and stored (frozen).
  Start making extra ice—maybe an ice mold if you're planning to use one.
  Discuss extra parking with neighbors if necessary.

Three to six days in advance
Begin decorating.
Make sure all is in order with your glassware, dishes, utensils.
   (If large ones are needed, borrow or rent.)

One to two days in advance
Buy perishables.
Purchase flowers and other fresh decorations.
Make extra room in the refrigerator by removing nonperishables to store elsewhere.
Make sure there is a place for guests' coats.
Check your tapes or CDs for appropriate music; you may need to borrow some.
Wash, clean, and cut vegetables and salad greens; store in individual plastic bags.
Make dips and/or salsa.

Day of party
Chill beverages early.
Finish food preparations.
Set out garbage cans.
Make sure all is in order in the bathroom.
Make sure there is a place for guests to put used dishes and glasses.
Set out some kind of outdoor decoration to identify your place for guests who have not been there before.
Time for your beauty treatment.
Welcome guests, make introductions, mingle, and enjoy.

Cooking for a Crowd

ITEM	12 SERVINGS	24 SERVINGS	48 SERVINGS
Punch	1½ quarts	3 quarts	1½ gallons
Iced tea	3 quarts	1½ gallons	3 gallons
Coffee			
(brewed)	9 cups	18 cups	36 cups
Cookies	2 dozen	4 dozen	8 dozen
Cakes			
9 x 13	1 cake	2 cakes	3 cakes
10-inch tube			
9-inch layer			
Tossed salad	4½ quarts	9 quarts	4½ gallons
Rolls	2 dozen	3 dozen	6 dozen
Meats			
(boneless)	3 pounds	6 pounds	12 pounds
Meats			
(bone in)	9 pounds	18 pounds	35 pounds
Cold cuts	2 pounds	4 pounds	8 pounds
Casseroles			
9 x 13	1 casserole	2 casseroles	4 casseroles
8-inch square	2 casseroles	4 casseroles	8 casseroles
Potato salad,			
coleslaw, or			
baked beans	1½ quarts	3 quarts	1½ gallons
Chicken salad	3 quarts	1½ gallons	3 gallons

The number of servings doesn't necessarily mean the number of guests served. Plan on one drink per hour per guest.

Fat Facts

SATURATED FATS: Most commonly found at room temperature. Most are in animal sources. Food products that are rich in saturated fats include meat, eggs, whole dairy products, some margarine and shortenings, coconut oil, and palm oil. These raise blood levels of total and LDL cholesterol.

UNSATURATED FATS: Found at room temperature; primary sources are plants. Polyunsaturated fats are highly unsaturated. Both types of unsaturated fats may help lower blood cholesterol levels when substituted for saturated fats. Food products high in polyunsaturated fats are corn oil, sunflower oil, soybean oil, safflower oil, and cottonseed oil. Oils high in monounsaturated fats are olive, canola, and peanut.

EXTRA LEAN: This means the product contains no more than 5 percent fat by weight. This does not apply to calories.

LOW-FAT: Yogurt and milk should contain between 0.5 and 2 percent milkfat to be labeled low-fat.

LOW-SODIUM: The product contains 140 milligrams of sodium or less per serving.

LOW-CALORIE: 40 calories or fewer per serving, or not more than 0.4 calorie per gram.

REDUCED-CALORIE: Product must contain ⅓ fewer calories than the food it replaces. Exceptions are meat and poultry products, which must contain ¼ fewer calories than similar products.

REDUCED-CHOLESTEROL: Product contains a 75 percent reduction of cholesterol.

Tips for Cutting the Fat

Fish: When baking fish, place rings of onion on the baking sheet, then lay the fish over the onion rings. This will prevent sticking and give a wonderful flavor to your fish.

Sauté means to fry quickly. Instead of sautéing in oil as most recipes call for, use ¼ cup of water instead, or try using chicken broth, rice vinegar, Worcestershire sauce, lime juice, or red wine vinegar. I save broth from veggies in a small container in the refrigerator to have something handy at all times without the expense.

Yogurt, non-fat: Try mixing a little Dijon mustard with some yogurt and using it instead of oil or mayonnaise to coat chicken or potato wedges before baking.

Yogurt the muffins. Use nonfat yogurt instead of oil in your muffins. Or use applesauce instead of oil.

Stuffing: When making stuffing from a two-step mix, substitute applesauce instead of margarine or butter. Nice flavor.

Mashed Potatoes: Try using skim buttermilk (1 fat gram per cup) instead of butter and milk, or just use skim milk and Butter Buds. You have the good butter flavor without the fat.

Hurry-up Potatoes: Mix 2 cups instant dried mashed potato flakes and ⅓ cup dried buttermilk powder, then add 2¾ cups boiling water. This makes about 4 cups of quick mashed, somewhat tangy potatoes.

Cut the amount of meat and increase the amount of vegetables in stews and soups.

There's the Beef: Try to take beef out of your diet as much as possible. You can substitute chicken or turkey in almost every recipe and never be unhappy with the flavor.

Sugar: You can reduce the amount of sugar in your baked goods by at least 1/3 and never know the difference. In all dishes except baked goods, you can use undiluted frozen apple juice, pears, bananas, or honey. Honey is sweeter and you will need less of it than you will of sugar.

Chocolate: Use 3 tablespoons of unsweetened cocoa powder and 1 tablespoon of polyunsaturated oil in place of each ounce of baking chocolate.

Cornstarch Trick: When using yogurt in hot dishes, add 1 teaspoon cornstarch for every cup of yogurt to keep it from separating on heating. If you are out of yogurt and in a hurry, blend 1 cup nonfat cottage cheese and 1 tablespoon of lemon juice with 2 tablespoons of skim milk. Try the cornstarch trick when using nonfat cream cheese also.

Fry Habit: Break the fry habit with broiling, roasting, baking, steaming, poaching, and stir-frying as your main cooking habit. Use the skillet for dry frying and sautéing but forget the oil.

Boil your stew meat or meat for your beans the day before and refrigerate the broth. The fat will congeal on the top. Next day, lift it off and go on with your recipe. You've still got the taste, and you've left the fat behind.

Trim any and all the fat you can possibly see from anything you are cooking. Saves you having to trim it from *you* later.

Eggs: I never use an egg anymore. You can use egg substitute—1/4 cup per 1 egg—in any recipe. You will never know the difference.

Salsa: Serving salsa is a good way to cut the fat. Use it instead of salad dressings to marinate chicken or fish, or serve it as a spicy side dish to curb the use of fatty sauces. Try it on your baked potato.

Extra: Cook a little extra of your fat-free meal and put into a divided microwave plate with a cover. Freeze, then take this to work instead of going out for lunch.

Switch to *fat-free* everything you can find on the market shelves. If you watch your fat intake you don't need to worry about counting your calories.

Water: Start every meal with a glass of water; this helps prevent overeating. Water is the best lubricant there is for your skin. It makes you pretty in more ways than one. Helps your complexion, helps your figure.

Weekends: Be good on weekends. Two days of overindulging can ruin five days of discipline. Make this low-fat eating a way of life, every day, all the time. Think low-fat. See what you can find and what you can eat—the markets are getting loaded with good low-fat products. There were none when I started; now it is a snap.

Substitutions

Living in Gore, Oklahoma, sometimes you find yourself short of an ingredient, but there are many substitutions you can make without ruining your dish.

Food Item	Substitute
2 tablespoons amaretto	¼–½ teaspoon almond extract
2 tablespoons Kahlúa or other coffee- or chocolate-flavored liqueur	½–1 teaspoon chocolate extract plus ½–1 teaspoon instant coffee in 2 tablespoons water
¼ cup or more red wine	Equal amount of red grape juice or cranberry juice
2 tablespoons rum or brandy	½–1 teaspoon rum or brandy extract, plus enough grape or apple juice to get correct amount of liquid needed for recipe
2 tablespoons sherry or bourbon	1–2 teaspoons vanilla extract
¼ cup or more port wine, sweet sherry, rum, brandy, or fruit-flavored liqueur	Equal amount of unsweetened orange or apple juice plus 1 teaspoon corresponding extract or vanilla extract
1 cup plain yogurt	1 cup low-fat buttermilk (1 gram per cup)
1 cup sour cream	1 cup fat-free yogurt plus 1 tablespoon cornstarch
1 cup buttermilk	1 cup skim milk plus 1 tablespoon white vinegar or lemon juice

1 cup milk	½ cup evaporated skim milk plus ½ cup water
1 pound mushrooms	1 (8-ounce) can sliced mushrooms, drained
1 small onion, chopped	1 tablespoon instant minced onion or 1 teaspoon onion powder
1 clove garlic, minced	⅛ teaspoon instant minced garlic or garlic powder
1 tablespoon chopped chives	1 tablespoon minced scallion tops
1 tablespoon grated fresh ginger	⅛ teaspoon ground ginger
1 tablespoon chopped dried orange peel	1½ teaspoons orange extract or 1 tablespoon grated fresh orange peel
1 (1-inch) piece vanilla bean	1 teaspoon vanilla extract
1 teaspoon ground allspice	½ teaspoon each ground cinnamon and ground cloves, mixed
1 teaspoon dry mustard	1 tablespoon prepared mustard
1 cup powdered sugar	1 cup granulated sugar plus 1 tablespoon cornstarch processed in food processor or blender
1 cup honey	1¼ cups sugar plus ⅓ cup water
1 cup pecans	1 cup regular oats, toasted (can use in baked products)
1 cup light corn syrup	1¼ cups sugar plus ⅓ cup water
1 cup tomato juice	½ cup tomato sauce plus ½ cup water
2 cups tomato sauce	¾ cup tomato paste plus 1 cup water

Seasoning Tips

Adding a dash of this and a pinch of that is expensive. I try not to use any spices and/or herbs that are not the commonly used regular-on-the-shelf type. Can't find those fancy out-of-the-ordinary spices in Gore, America, anyway.

SHOPPING

Look for bottles or jars with screw-top lids or tins with tight-fitting lids. These types are more airtight.

Shop at large stores that continually restock the shelves. "Old" seasonings with a dull color are safe to use but don't have much flavor.

Purchase dried herbs and spices in small amounts. Once opened, they begin to deteriorate after three months if not stored properly.

For maximum flavor, purchase whole spices and crush small amounts with a mortar and pestle, meat mallet, or rolling pin, or even the bottom of a cast-iron skillet. Grind larger amounts in a pepper mill, coffee grinder, or blender.

STORAGE

Store dried seasonings in a cool, dry, dark place. Protection from heat, moisture, and strong light is essential.

Don't display seasonings on open racks above or near stovetops, ovens, or dishwashers. Heat speeds their deterioration.

Store dried whole spices and herbs in the freezer for up to three years. Store ground seasonings in the freezer for up to six months.

Record the date of purchase with a permanent marker on the container.

Check for a change in color, a musty odor, or a faint aroma. These indicate a spice that is past its prime. Doubling the amount will not make up the difference or loss in flavor.

GARLIC

Select firm heads with plump outside cloves and no noticeable sprouting or dark spots. The flavor of sprouted garlic is harsh. If it must be used, cut the clove in half and remove the center green-colored sprout.

Crushed, minced, or pressed garlic is more intense than garlic cloves that are halved, sliced, or left whole.

Press a clove through a garlic press with the peel left on in order to produce maximum flavor and leave hands odor free. To remove garlic odor from hands, rub them first with lemon juice, then salt; rinse and wash next with soap.

To peel, place the flat side of a chef's knife blade on top of the garlic clove and hit it with your fist. The blow separates the papery skin from the clove for easy removal.

Store whole heads of garlic in a cool, dark, well-ventilated place up to eight weeks. Once broken from the head, individual cloves will keep up to about ten days.

Garlic yields: 1 medium clove garlic equals ½ teaspoon minced fresh or ½ teaspoon minced from a jar or ⅛ teaspoon garlic powder or instant minced garlic.

Source: *America's Best Recipes*

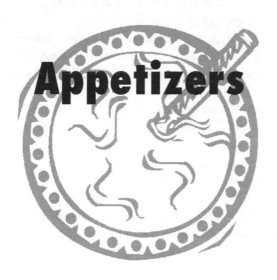

Appetizers

COUNTRY CAVIAR

In the country, we use cornmeal for every-thing. What you have is what you use, so make something with what you have.

SERVES 12

VERY LOW-FAT

Prep :10
Cook :15
Stand :00
Total :25

1¼ cups fat-free self-rising cornmeal mix
¼ cup egg substitute
½ cup fat-free sour cream
½ teaspoon chopped chives (fresh or dried)
24 pitted ripe or pimento-stuffed olives

Preheat the oven to 400 degrees. Lightly spray two miniature (1¾-inch) muffin pans with vegetable oil cooking spray.

In a heavy zipper-lock plastic bag, combine cornmeal mix, egg substitute, sour cream, and chives. Close the bag and use tips of fingers to mix batter well. Keep walking your fingers around and over the batter until well blended. Shake to one side of the bag and snip off the corner of the bag to make a ¾-inch opening. Squeeze the batter into the prepared muffin pans, filling each about ¾ full.

Press an olive into the center of each cup of batter. Bake for about 15 minutes or until done.

Variations: Use cocktail onions or a ring of jalapeño pepper in place of the olives.

Make a thumbprint in the top of each cup of batter and spoon in about ½ teaspoon of minced fresh jalapeño pepper, or jalapeño pepper jelly.

Variations: Add a ½-inch chunk of fat-free cheese, your choice.
Add a ½-inch chunk of 98% fat-free ham.
Add ¼ teaspoon of hot pepper sauce.

HOT AND SPICY PEPPER SQUARES

½ cup flour
1 teaspoon baking powder
Dash salt
2 cups egg substitute
3 cups grated fat-free Monterey Jack cheese
1½ cups fat-free cottage cheese
2 tablespoons chopped pickled jalapeño pepper
2 tablespoons chopped pimento
2 tablespoons sliced pitted ripe olives

MAKES 48
SQUARES

0 GRAMS FAT

Prep :10
Cook :40
Stand :10
Total 1:00

Preheat the oven to 350 degrees. Lightly spray a 13 x 9-inch baking dish with vegetable oil cooking spray.

In a bowl stir together the flour, baking powder, and salt. Set aside.

In a large mixing bowl, beat the egg substitute slightly with an electric mixer, then stir in the flour mixture. Fold in the cheeses, pepper, pimento, and olives.

Pour into the prepared baking dish. Bake uncovered for about 40 minutes, or until set and golden brown. Let stand 10 minutes; cut into 1½-inch squares. Serve warm or with low-fat tortilla chips if desired.

FROZEN GRAPES

1½ pounds green or red seedless grapes

SERVES 6

0 GRAMS FAT

Prep :50
Cook :00
Stand :02
Total :52

Stem and wash the grapes and pat dry. Place in the freezer for about 45 minutes. Remove from the freezer and let stand 2 minutes before serving.

Very good with a hot spicy meal on a hot spicy summer evening.

BEAN TASTIES

MAKES 40 TASTIES

2.3 GRAMS FAT PER SERVING (4 PIECES)

Prep :20
Cook :10
Stand :00
Total :30

½ cup chopped onion
1 (16-ounce) can fat-free refried beans
½ cup salsa
1 teaspoon chili powder
⅛ teaspoon garlic powder
Dash salt (optional)
Dash pepper
¼ cup fat-free cream cheese, at room temperature
½ cup cubed avocado
1 teaspoon lime juice
1 teaspoon lemon juice
10 (6-inch) flour tortillas
½ cup finely chopped green peppers (or red or mixed for holidays)
Salsa and fat-free sour cream

In a nonstick skillet lightly sprayed with vegetable oil cooking spray, cook the onion, stirring constantly, until tender. Stir in the refried beans, salsa, chili powder, garlic powder, salt, if desired, and pepper. Set aside.

Combine the cream cheese, avocado, and lime and lemon juice and mash together thoroughly. Spread about 2 tablespoons over each tortilla, leaving about ½-inch border around edge. Spread about 2 tablespoons of the bean mixture over the avocado mixture. Top with a chopped pepper and roll each tortilla up.

Cut the tortilla rolls into fourths; insert a toothpick or wooden pick into each tastie. Serve with salsa and fat-free sour cream.

HAM SWIRLS

8 slices 98% fat-free deli-style ham
1 (8-ounce) package fat-free cream cheese, at room temperature
8 medium whole dill pickles

Spread one side of each ham slice with about 2 tablespoons of cream cheese.

Lay one pickle on each at one side; roll the ham slice around the pickle. Press the edges together. Cover and refrigerate 1 hour. To serve, cut each pickle into six slices. Place on a serving tray, flat side down. Have picks by the tray.

SERVES 8

1 GRAM FAT
PER SERVING

Prep :15
Cook :00
Stand 1:00
Total 1:15

PIZZA APPETIZERS

1 long loaf Italian bread, cut in half lengthwise
¾ cup shredded fat-free Monterey Jack cheese
¾ cup shredded fat-free Cheddar Cheese
¾ cup fat-free pasta sauce
1½ tablespoons dried Italian seasoning
6 thin slices 98% fat-free ham
12 to 15 bell pepper rings
½ cup chopped onion
Parsley for garnish

Preheat the broiler. Place the bread, cut side up, on a baking sheet; toast 4 to 5 inches from the heat source until lightly browned.

Combine the cheeses and sprinkle ¼ of the mixture on each bread half; broil again until the cheese melts, about 1 to 2 minutes.

In a small saucepan, combine the pasta sauce and seasoning. Place over medium heat until thoroughly heated. Spoon evenly over bread halves; top with ham, pepper rings, and chopped onion. Sprinkle each half with the remaining cheeses. *(continued)*

SERVES 12

2 GRAMS FAT
PER SERVING

Prep :15
Cook :08
Stand :00
Total :23

Broil 4 to 5 minutes or until the cheese is melted. Cut each half into 6 pieces. Garnish with a little parsley if desired.

TORTILLA CHEESECAKE

SERVES 12

2 GRAMS FAT
ENTIRE DISH

Prep :35
Cook :45
Stand 3:00
Total 4:20

1½ cups crushed baked tortilla chips
¼ cup Butter Buds, liquid form
2 (8-ounce) packages plus 1 (3-ounce) package fat-free cream cheese, at room
    temperature
½ cup egg substitute
2½ cups shredded fat-free Monterey Jack cheese
1 (4-ounce) can chopped green chiles, drained
¼ teaspoon ground red pepper (cayenne)
1 (8-ounce) carton fat-free sour cream
1½ cups chopped bell peppers
½ cup chopped scallions
1 medium tomato, chopped

Preheat the oven to 325 degrees. Lightly spray the bottom of a 9-inch springform pan with vegetable oil cooking spray.

Process the crushed tortilla chips into fine crumbs in a blender or food processor. Or place the chips in a zipper-lock plastic bag and roll into crumbs with a rolling pin or bottle.

Combine the crushed tortilla chips with the Butter Buds and mix well. Press onto the bottom of the springform pan. Bake for 15 minutes and let cool on a wire rack.

Stir the cream cheese gently with a wire whisk. Add the egg substitute slowly, mixing after each addition. Stir in the shredded cheeses, chiles, and ground red pepper. Pour into the prepared pan, and bake at 325 degrees for 30 minutes. Cool 10 minutes on a wire rack. Gently run a knife around the edge of the pan to release the sides, and let cool completely.

Spread the sour cream evenly over the top; cover and chill. Arrange the chopped peppers and chopped scallions over the top and the tomatoes around the edge of top as desired. During the holidays I make mine in the shape of a tree.

Serve with tortilla chips.

CHILES RELLENOS

6 ounces fat-free Monterey Jack cheese
3 (4-ounce) cans whole green chiles, drained and seeded
½ cup all-purpose flour
⅛ teaspoon salt
⅛ teaspoon pepper
¼ cup egg substitute
1 (14-ounce) can stewed tomatoes, undrained and chopped

SERVES 4

LOW-FAT

Prep :25
Cook :40
Stand :00
Total 1:05

Preheat the oven to 350 degrees. Lightly spray a 13 x 9-inch baking dish with vegetable oil cooking spray.

Cut the cheese into pieces; place one piece inside each chile. (You may use shredded cheese.) Set the cheese-filled chiles aside.

Combine the flour, salt, and pepper in a small mixing bowl. Place the egg substitute in another small bowl. Dredge each chile in the flour, then dip in the egg substitute. In a nonstick skillet lightly sprayed with vegetable oil cooking spray, brown the chiles.

Transfer the browned chiles to the prepared baking dish. Pour undrained chopped tomatoes over chiles. Bake for 30 minutes.

Serve with Mexican meals.

PITA PIZZA SNACKS

1 fat-free pita bread, split into 2 rounds
2 tablespoons fat-free Italian dressing
2 slices fat-free cheese
Pizza toppings: chopped onions, peppers, sliced mushrooms

SERVES 2

0 GRAMS FAT

Prep :10
Cook :12
Stand :00
Total :22

Preheat the oven to 375 degrees. Lightly brush the pita bread with dressing, place on a baking sheet, and bake for 8 to 10 minutes or until lightly browned. Brush bread with half of the remaining dressing; top with cheese and desired toppings. Drizzle the remaining dressing over the top. Return to the oven and bake for an additional 1 or 2 minutes, or until cheese begins to melt. Cut each round into 8 wedges.

MINI BAGEL BITS

SERVES 4

0.5 GRAM FAT PER BAGEL (2 HALVES)

Prep :10
Cook :08
Stand :00
Total :18

8 mini bagels, sliced in half
Fat-free pizza sauce
½ cup chopped onion
½ cup chopped bell pepper
1 cup shredded fat-free mozzarella or Cheddar cheese or both

Preheat the oven to 400 degrees. Place the bagels cut side up on a baking sheet. Spread the desired amount of pizza sauce on each bagel half. Top with onion, pepper, and cheese. Bake for about 7 to 8 minutes, until the bagels are hot and the cheese is melted.

HOLIDAY POPCORN SPECIAL

SERVES 5

0 GRAMS FAT

Prep :15
Cook :15
Stand :00
Total :30

1 egg white
2 tablespoons packed brown sugar or Brown Sugar Twin
⅛ teaspoon cinnamon
3 quarts (12 cups) air-popped popcorn

Preheat the oven to 325 degrees. Lightly spray a 15 x 10-inch baking pan with vegetable oil cooking spray.

In a small bowl, beat the egg white until soft peaks form. Add the brown sugar or Sugar Twin and cinnamon, beating until stiff peaks form (usually about 1 minute). Place popcorn in a large bowl. Fold the egg white mixture into the popcorn. Spread in prepared baking sheet. Bake for 15 minutes, stirring twice during baking. Cool completely. Store in an airtight container.

Variations: Substitute 2 tablespoons barbecue seasoning for the sugar and cinnamon. If you like spicy snacks, substitute Cajun seasoning for the sugar and cinnamon.

WHITE BEAN DIP

2 (16-ounce) cans Great Northern beans
1 (4-ounce) can chopped green chiles
¼ cup salsa
2 tablespoons lemon juice
½ clove garlic, minced
Pinch of dried basil
2 scallions, chopped fine
4 to 6 drops hot pepper sauce (careful—add 1 drop at a time)

SERVES 4

0 GRAMS FAT

Prep :10
Cook :00
Stand 1:00
Total 1:10

Drain the beans and chiles. Place in a food processor or blender, add the salsa, lemon juice, garlic, and basil. Blend until smooth.

Remove from the container into a mixing bowl. Stir in the scallions—this will give a little body and crunch to your dip. Add hot pepper sauce a couple drops at a time, tasting frequently. Chill about an hour before serving.

SALSA DIP

1 (8-ounce) package fat-free cream cheese, at room temperature
½ cup spicy salsa
2 to 3 drops hot pepper sauce

SERVES 4

0 GRAMS FAT

Prep :05
Cook :00
Stand :00
Total :05

In a small mixing bowl, stir all the above ingredients together with a wire whisk. Be gentle with the stirring of the cream cheese; fat-free cheese gets thin very easily. Add only one drop of hot sauce at a time until the temperature suits your taste.

VEGETABLE DIP

SERVES 8

0 GRAMS FAT

Prep :20
Cook :00
Stand 3:00
Total 3:20

1 head cauliflower
1 bunch broccoli
1 (16-ounce) bag carrots
2 (8-ounce) packages fat-free cream cheese, at room temperature
½ cup minced onion
½ teaspoon ground cumin
¼ teaspoon chili powder
Dash of salt
8 to 10 drops hot pepper sauce
Dippers: broccoli, cauliflower florets, carrots, celery, cucumber sticks, low-fat chips

Break cauliflower and broccoli into florets. Mince 1 cup of each and reserve remainder for dippers. Mince ½ cup carrots very tiny; cut remainder into small sticks for dippers.

In a medium mixing bowl, blend cream cheese (stir very gently—fat-free cream cheese breaks down easily) with onion and seasonings. Add the hot pepper sauce one drop at a time, tasting after each addition. Stir in the minced cauliflower, broccoli, and carrots. Refrigerate in a covered bowl at least 3 hours or overnight before serving. Crackers are also nice dippers.

ZIPPY DIP

SERVES 8

0 GRAMS FAT

Prep :15
Cook :00
Stand 3:00
Total 3:15

2 (8-ounce) packages fat-free cream cheese, at room temperature
½ cup spicy V-8 vegetable juice
1 (4-ounce) can chopped green chiles, drained
¼ cup chopped bell pepper
¼ cup minced onion
4 drops hot pepper sauce
Fresh vegetables for dippers

In a medium bowl with a wire whisk, gently stir the cream cheese until smooth. (Careful—fat-free cream cheese can break down and get runny.) Gradually add V-8 juice until smooth and well blended.

Stir in chiles, pepper, onion, and pepper sauce one drop at a time, tasting after each, to be sure you don't get it too hot. Cover and refrigerate at least 3 hours.

This is a good make-ahead dip.

SPINACH DIP

1 (10-ounce) package frozen chopped spinach, thawed
1 (8-ounce) can water chestnuts, drained and chopped
1 (16-ounce) carton fat-free sour cream
½ cup fat-free salad dressing
1 (8-ounce) envelope vegetable soup mix
½ teaspoon lemon juice

MAKES
ABOUT 3
CUPS

0 GRAMS FAT

Prep :15
Cook :00
Stand 1:00
Total 1:15

Drain thawed spinach on paper towels, squeezing out liquid. Combine spinach, water chestnuts, and remaining ingredients; cover and chill for 1 hour. Serve with assorted fresh vegetables.

GUACAMOLE THE SLIM WAY

1 (20-ounce) bag frozen green peas, thawed and drained
¼ cup lime juice
2 tablespoons chopped fresh cilantro or 1 teaspoon dried
½ small onion, quartered
2 tablespoons chopped green chiles
¼ cup picante sauce or salsa
Salt and pepper to taste
1 small fresh tomato, chopped into tiny pieces

SERVES 6

0 GRAMS FAT

Prep :15
Cook :00
Stand :00
Total :15

In a blender or food processor, process peas, lime juice, cilantro, onion, and chiles until smooth. Transfer to a mixing bowl and stir in picante sauce, salt and pepper, and chopped tomato. Stir together. Serve with Tortilla Chips (page 39).

CREAMY DIP

**MAKES
ABOUT 1
CUP**

0 GRAMS FAT

**Prep :05
Cook :00
Stand 2:00
Total 2:05**

½ cup fat-free sour cream
½ cup fat-free mayonnaise
1 tablespoon chopped chives
1½ tablespoons Worcestershire sauce
½ teaspoon seasoned salt

In a mixing bowl, combine all ingredients and blend thoroughly. Cover the mixture and chill for a couple of hours before serving, letting flavors blend.

Serve the dip with assorted fresh vegetables and chips.

SWEET POTATO CHIPS

SERVES 4

**TRACE OF FAT
PER SERVING**

**Prep :10
Cook :25
Stand :00
Total :35**

2 large sweet potatoes, peeled
¼ teaspoon salt (optional)

Preheat the oven to 325 degrees. Lightly spray two baking sheets with vegetable oil cooking spray.

Using a very sharp knife or vegetable cutter, slice the sweet potatoes crosswise into ⅛-inch slices. Arrange in a single layer on the prepared baking sheets. Lightly coat the slices with cooking spray.

Bake for 15 to 25 minutes or until crisp. Remove the chips from baking sheets as they begin to brown. Cool; sprinkle with salt if desired. Store in an airtight container.

TATER DIPPERS

4 to 5 cups raw vegetables (mushrooms, bell peppers, broccoli, carrots; see below)
1 cup instant potato flakes
⅓ cup grated fat-free Parmesan cheese
½ teaspoon celery salt
¼ teaspoon garlic powder
½ cup egg substitute
Fat-free ranch salad dressing (fat-free) or dip (optional)

SERVES 6

0 GRAMS FAT

Prep :10
Cook :25
Stand :00
Total :35

Preheat the oven to 400 degrees. Lightly spray two baking sheets with vegetable oil cooking spray.

Prepare the vegetables: Wipe the mushrooms and leave them whole. Core the peppers and cut into rings. Separate the broccoli into florets. Peel the carrots and cut into thin strips.

In a small bowl, combine the potato flakes, Parmesan cheese, celery salt, and garlic powder. In another bowl, beat the egg substitute slightly. Dip the vegetables, one at a time, in the egg substitute, then in the potato mixture. Arrange them on the prepared baking sheets and spray lightly with vegetable oil cooking spray. Bake for 20 to 25 minutes, until tender. Serve with dressing or dip if desired, or you can just use as your vegetable side dish.

TORTILLA CHIPS

Multiply as needed for number of servings.

1 flour tortilla or corn tortilla

SERVES 1

1 GRAM FAT
PER 8 CHIPS

Prep :05
Cook :15
Stand :00
Total :20

Preheat the oven to 350 degrees.

Lightly spray the corn tortilla, if using, with a fine mist of water (flour tortillas don't need any preparation). Cut into 8 wedge-shape pieces, place on a baking sheet, and bake until lightly browned, about 10 to 15 minutes. Be careful to watch what you're doing; they will burn very quickly.

Soups and Salads

GARDEN SOUP

SERVES 8

**1 GRAM FAT
PER 2-CUP
SERVING**

**Prep :25
Cook 1:15
Stand :00
Total 1:40**

8 boneless, skinless chicken tenders
1 bell pepper, seeded and chopped
2 banana peppers, seeded and chopped
1 large onion, chopped
4 ears corn, kernels cut off the cob (about 2 cups)
1½ cups frozen peas and carrots
1 cup chopped celery
4 medium potatoes, peeled and cubed
Salt and pepper to taste
½ teaspoon oregano
½ teaspoon basil
2 drops Tabasco
¼ teaspoon adobo seasoning (optional)
2 cups sliced okra (½-inch pieces)
1 tablespoon vinegar
1½ cups uncooked rigatoni
1½ cups chopped cabbage

Bring 2 quarts of water to a boil in a large saucepan or soup kettle. Add the chicken tenders, lower the heat, and simmer until cooked through, 15 to 20 minutes. Remove the chicken with a slotted spoon. When cool enough to handle, cut into bite-size pieces and set aside.

Meantime, to the boiling chicken stock add the chopped peppers, onion, corn, peas and carrots, celery, and potatoes. Add a little more water to replace what has boiled away. Season with salt, pepper, oregano, basil, and Tabasco, and the adobo if desired. Bring to a boil over high heat, lower the heat to medium, and simmer until tender, about 20 minutes.

In a small saucepan, cover the okra with water, add 1 tablespoon vinegar (this keeps it from being slimy), and boil until tender, 3 to 4 minutes. Drain and rinse; set aside. In a separate saucepan, boil rigatoni according to package directions, drain, and rinse; set aside.

When the veggies are almost tender, add the okra, rigatoni, cabbage, and chicken. Continue cooking until done to desired tenderness.

Serve with dry-fried cornbread cakes.

BROCCOLI SOUP

4 cups chopped fresh broccoli (about 1½ pounds)
1 cup chopped celery
1 cup chopped carrots
¾ cup chopped onion
2¼ cups skim milk
¼ cup flour
4 cups fat-free chicken broth
½ teaspoon minced fresh parsley
1 teaspoon onion salt
Dash garlic powder
Salt and pepper to taste
2 teaspoons cornstarch (optional)
¼ cup cold skim milk (optional)

SERVES 6

0 GRAMS FAT

Prep :20
Cook :40
Stand :00
Total 1:00

In your favorite soup kettle or deep dutch oven, bring 4 cups of water to a boil. Drop in the broccoli, celery, carrots, and half the onions. Boil for 3 to 4 minutes, drain in a colander in the sink, and set aside.

In the same pan, sauté the remaining onions in ¼ cup water until tender (watch closely—you may need to add a little more water if it cooks dry). Add ¼ cup of the skim milk, bring to a simmer, and stir in the flour to form a smooth paste. Gradually add the chicken broth and the remaining 2 cups milk, stirring constantly. Bring to a boil over medium heat and stir for 1 minute.

Add the vegetables, parsley, and seasonings. Reduce the heat to low and simmer for 30 to 40 minutes or until the vegetables are tender. Be careful not to burn; keep the heat regulated to low.

When vegetables have reached the desired degree of doneness, cover the pan and turn the heat off. Just before serving you may want to thicken your soup a little with the cornstarch and ¼ cup cold skim milk. Mix these together, return the soup to boiling, and stir in the cornstarch mixture a little at a time until soup thickens.

CREAMY CORN CHOWDER

Corn holds a special place in our family, as it was always Dad's favorite. He would say, "This must be Sloan corn." My brother grows sweet corn and field corn. Best in the world, bar none.

SERVES 4

LESS THAN 1 GRAM FAT PER SERVING

Prep :20
Cook :15
Stand :00
Total :35

4 ears fresh corn or 1 (10-ounce) package frozen whole-kernel corn
¾ to 1 cup peeled and cubed potatoes (small cubes)
½ cup chopped onion
½ cup thinly sliced celery
1 teaspoon instant chicken bouillon granules
Dash pepper (white looks better but black is fine)
1¾ cups skim milk
2 tablespoons flour
2 tablespoons nonfat dry milk powder

If using fresh corn, cut the kernels off with a sharp knife; you should have about 2 cups of corn. In a large saucepan, combine the corn, potatoes, onion, celery, bouillon granules, pepper, and ⅓ cup water. Bring to a boil, lower the heat, and simmer for about 10 minutes or until the corn and potatoes are just tender. Stir often. Stir in 1½ cups of the milk. Continue to cook on low heat until the milk has become hot.

In a separate bowl, combine the flour and dry milk powder. Stir in the remaining ¼ cup of skim milk with a wire whisk, stirring until smooth. Gradually add to the corn mixture, stirring carefully so as not to mash your vegetables, until thickened. Cook about 1 minute more on low heat, being careful not to burn.

Serve in soup bowls, garnished with bacon bits if desired. Makes 4 servings, or 2 servings if this is your main dish; serve with a nice salad.

WHITE BEAN SOUP

2 cups dried Great Northern beans
2 tablespoons instant chicken bouillon granules
½ teaspoon salt (optional)
1 medium onion, chopped
1 clove garlic, minced
1 medium carrot, sliced
1 stalk celery, sliced
1 medium potato, peeled and diced
1 tablespoon chopped fresh parsley

SERVES 6

0.5 GRAMS FAT PER 1½-CUP SERVING

Prep :15
Cook 2:15
Stand :00
Total 2:30

Look over and wash the beans thoroughly. Place in a deep stock-pot, add 6 cups of water, and bring to a boil. Boil for about 5 minutes, then reduce heat to a simmer. Add the bouillon, salt, if desired, onion, and garlic. Simmer for 1 to 1½ hours, until the beans are tender. Remove 2 cups of bean mixture, purée in a food processor, and return the puréed beans to the stockpot. Add the carrot, celery, and potato.

Cover and simmer an additional 30 to 45 minutes, or until the vegetables are tender. Just before serving, stir in the parsley.

AFTER-THE-HOLIDAYS
TURKEY AND BEAN SOUP

SERVES 6

**2–3 GRAMS
FAT PER 1½-
CUP SERVING**

**Prep :25
Cook 2:00
Stand :00
Total 2:25**

2 cups chopped cooked turkey (left over from the holidays)
1 (16-ounce) can stewed tomatoes
1 (14-ounce) can pinto beans, drained
1 (12-ounce) can Great Northern beans, drained
1 (14-ounce) can whole-kernel corn
1 cup chopped onion
6 rings jalapeño peppers, chopped
2 cloves garlic, minced
2 (16-ounce) cans fat-free chicken broth
1 (12-ounce) can light beer
3 tablespoons chili powder
1 teaspoon dried basil
1 teaspoon thyme leaves
¼ teaspoon pepper

In a large dutch oven (I use a cast-iron dutch oven on my wood stove), combine all ingredients. Bring to a boil over medium heat. Reduce the heat and simmer, uncovered, for about 2 hours. Stir occasionally.

This is very nice after the holidays to just dump all in one cookpot, using up some of that leftover turkey, and set it on the wood stove to simmer as you spend a long winter day undecorating, sewing, or whatever you like. Serve with a pone of cornbread. The aroma of this cooking all day will drive you crazy.

DAD'S GARDEN

I have many harrowing as well as happy memories of Dad's gardens. My earliest memory of the garden was when I was five years old. All four of us—Dad, Mom, Brother, and I—were down in the garden picking English peas (you may call them green peas). I had a very loose front tooth. I was pestering my dad, flitting around wiggling this terrible-looking loose tooth, all the while being warned by him that he was getting a little weary of my snaggle tooth and he was just about to pull it out.

My grandmother, his mother, lived just down the way, and you know how little girls are about their grandmothers. She was just the berries. I smart-mouthed one time too many as he warned me about pulling this tooth. I remember saying, "No you won't. I'll tell Ma Sloan on you!"

Too late! I was flat on my back in the middle of the pea row and my tooth was gone! I can still remember running down the road, yelling, "Ma! Ma!," blood just trickling but it seemed to me that it was gushing. "Daddy pulled my tooth! Daddy pulled my tooth! Ma! Ma!"

I remember the warmth of those old wrinkled arms wrapped around me to comfort my disbelief that a smart remark could have this result. I can still see that old apron she always wore—she carried vegetables in it cupped up like a basket. There is real magic in a grandma's arms, especially when you need protection from a parent.

He never followed me, or said another word about the tooth. None needed. I never smart-mouthed my dad or threatened him with a grandparent again, ever. Lesson well learned, quick.

Dad, being a farmer, with large fields, never believed in just planting a regular-size garden, like 30 by 50 or so. He always planted a garden about an acre or sometimes 1½ acres. He wanted to be sure everyone had veggies out of his wonderful gardens. He did have the best one in town. My brother and I always got on the end of the long rows, helping to plant sixty, eighty, a hundred tomato plants, planting 200 pounds of potatoes—four to six rows—all the way through the garden of okra. Do you have any idea how much okra was ready to be picked off those long rows every other day? Bob and I would go and pick five or six 5-gallon buckets full of okra. Good grief! What do you do with that much okra? There weren't enough people in the little town of Gore to eat that much okra. I always felt like the Little Red Hen. I would ask if anyone at church wanted any okra. No one, unless you picked it and brought it to them. To say yes, we will come and pick it, was just out of the question.

Dad's gardens were wonderful, but work! Oh, the heat, sweat, dust, bugs . . . and when it was picked, that was just the beginning for me. Dad would get his feelings hurt if you didn't want vegetables, and if no one put them up. Mom used to, but in her later years—the past ten—she didn't, so guess who that left. You got it: me! Sometimes I would go home with five or six 5-gallon buckets of tomatoes to can, five or six 5-gallon buckets of okra to freeze, squash by the basketsful, peppers to freeze—all with Dad to please.

I have a golf cart with a red wagon that we pull behind it for gardening and yard work. Sometimes the cart wouldn't hardly make it over the pond bank between Dad's house and our house. This pond is the fish pond, but I'll make that another story.

This year is the second time I have had my own garden since I have moved back to the country. The first one was the year the house was finished, but we still lived in Tulsa, just coming on the weekends. It was laid out just the way Dad would do it—big. I think maybe he might have had a hand in doing that. Needless to say, we couldn't keep up with it, and not being here every day, with just weekends to work on it, it wasn't enough. We wound up mowing it with an 11-horsepower tractor. That was the end of our gardening on our own for a few years. It was enough just to keep up a five-acre yard.

This spring my brother came over one Sunday afternoon—late, just about five. Bob and I had been working outside, and we'd showered and retired for the evening. *Not!* He said, I think I'll make you a raised bed garden like mine, okay? Well, you don't look a gift horse in the mouth, even though the thoughts were going through my head: I don't want a garden. (I find it too easy to go to Sarge's, a local vegetable stand). What in the world will I do with a garden. Oh, my.

"Oh, that will be nice, thank you."

He said, "I'm going to get my tractor. I'll be back in a minute."

"Okay."

He lived just up the way from me, about half a mile. I commented to Bob, "Guess what? I'm getting a garden." About 15 minutes went by. I thought he was going over to get my nephew's little John Deere that he uses to mow the pasture with, etc. Faint I almost did when he turned into our drive with this tractor that he does his farm with. It is so big, you just can't imagine. It is a long piece of machinery that you cut out dirt with and haul it off. He made a long cut down through my beautiful green lawn, over by the little house and shed. For a raised bed garden, you build up the dirt and build a frame around it. He took out three loads of my poor soil and brought some good soil from some land we have a short ways off. Five loads. It sure looks like a big pile of dirt.

Well, you guessed it, now poor Bob gets to go to work. The next day he had me go over to the lumber yard and order up treated lumber for him to frame it up with—12 inches wide, so the garden is raised 12 inches. I got lumber, $236; nails, $3.45; black soil cloth (cloth you put on top of your flower bed, for instance to keep grass from growing), $23; 50 bags of cedar chips, $185.76; bedding plants, $27.48; fertilizer, $12; a proper tool, $10.95—so far, my little 12-foot-wide and 55-foot-long garden has cost me $498.64 and the frame is not even around it yet.

For the next three days, Bob came home and went straight to the garden to work, driving stakes into the ground to nail the frame with—oops, we didn't get enough lumber, another $137 ($635.64 update). Now, you can't appreciate this man I am married to unless I elaborate to you just a little. He drives for 1 hour and 15 minutes, about 75 miles, to work each day—leaves home at 6:00 A.M. and returns around 6:30 P.M. With Daylight Saving Time, he could put in some pretty good licks on that pile of lumber. Bless his heart. He doesn't mess around once I get him started. In just about four days, it was finished. All this time, from the time he left until he returned, I would be working on the top of this little vegetable patch. Leveling the dirt, putting down the black cloth, spreading the chips—oops, we didn't get enough 40-pound bags of cedar chips. Another $58 ($693.64 update).

After about seven days of continuous work, we had a pretty good-looking garden. I almost had it full with nice pretty little plants— tomatoes, peppers, squash, okra, and oh, yes, no lady should have a garden without flowers. I put flowers across the end and all down both sides at the end of each row. My brother asked me how I was going to cook those red things, and I simply said, "Stir-fry."

I was walking down the back of the yard, where we have an area that we store things in—you know those kinds of things: leftover lumber, leftover bricks . . . Look. Bricks. I know what, I could build myself a little wall around the garden, which would make it a foot larger. I could plant my peppers and things there. Yes! I will build myself a brick wall and it will look nice from the drive as you come in.

I have this man, Carey, who has worked for me for years. His mother worked for my mother. He has moved these bricks from one place to another at least six times. I will call Carey to come and help me. "Hello, Carey, I have this little chore I would like for you to come to help me do." "Okay." He arrives. What is the job? Oh, would you please move the brick from down in the draw up to the garden. I thought he was just going to go get into that old blue Jeep truck he has and run over me, but he laughed and said, "Okay." Bless you, Carey. Fifty-five dollars for Carey. Update: $748.64.

For the next three days, I mixed cement and laid my brick wall, three bricks high. Cement, $4.36. Update: $753. By this time it is beginning to look like the Great Wall of China. I think I'll stop with the end next to the drive and the side next to the drive. Looks pretty sharp. Now all I need is just the right flowers: $36. Update: $789 for this little garden with the brick wall. Did just that: I put the brick holes up and put some potting soil, $16 ($805 update), in the holes, planted little plants in the holes. Wish you could see this lady-looking beautiful garden, and so far the pleasure has been all mine.

I must say, I was really starting to enjoy my little garden. I would spend just about every day out there. I did *not* have one weed in it. I fertilized, watered, planted, and was so proud. It was really growing. I was amazed, most of all at the pleasure I was getting out of this. I thanked my brother several times, even though I was reluctant at first.

My garden was very productive. I definitely am looking forward to planting another one next year. After all, how many vegetables could I have bought for $805? Ha! Not on your life. Today I had to pay Carey to clean out the garden, haul off all the dead vines, pull the tomato stakes out, etc. Next season will be here before we know it, and the cycle starts all over, except the building part is done and paid for, so it won't be so bad again.

I could not believe how many vegetables I did get out of this garden. I gave veggies to everyone. I have retired my canning days—eat it, freeze it, or give it away.

Garden-day memories will never leave me. Every time I do anything out there it reminds me of the days I spent with Dad in his gardens. I can still see him walking from the back of the house down to the garden.

Amen!

Dad died August 10, 1995.

VEGETABLE SALAD

A good do-ahead recipe for entertaining.

SERVES 6

0 GRAMS FAT

Prep :10
Cook :00
Stand 3:00
Total 3:10

2 cups broccoli florets
2 cups cauliflower florets
6 large mushrooms, sliced
1 small onion, sliced
¼ cup sliced celery
½ cup fat-free honey mustard salad dressing
¼ cup white vinegar
1 tablespoon poppy seeds
½ teaspoon salt (optional)

In a large mixing bowl, combine the broccoli, cauliflower, mushrooms, onion, and celery. In a small mixing bowl, combine the salad dressing, vinegar, poppy seeds, and salt if using. Mix with a wire whisk. Pour over the vegetables and toss to coat evenly.

Cover and chill for 3 hours, stirring occasionally. Serve with a slotted spoon.

TASTY TOMATO SLICES

SERVES 6

1 GRAM FAT
PER SERVING

Prep :10
Cook :00
Stand 2:00
Total 2:10

3 medium tomatoes, cut into ¼-inch slices
¼ cup wine vinegar (use tarragon if available)
1 teaspoon canola oil
1 tablespoon chopped fresh tarragon leaves or 1 teaspoon dried
Fresh ground pepper

Place the tomatoes in a glass or plastic container, or a serving dish. Shake the vinegar, oil, and tarragon in a jar to mix well. Pour over tomatoes. Sprinkle with pepper and cover. Refrigerate for at least 2 hours.

This serves as a quick salad and can be made ahead.

MARINATED COLESLAW

6 cups shredded cabbage
1 large onion, sliced thin and separated into rings
½ cup sugar
½ cup cider vinegar
1 tablespoon canola oil
¼ teaspoon garlic salt
¼ teaspoon pepper
¼ teaspoon celery seed

SERVES 8

2 GRAMS FAT PER SERVING

Prep :15
Cook :00
Stand 6:00
Total 6:15

In a large container with a cover (Tupperware-type bowl) place the shredded cabbage and onion rings. Toss to mix. In a small bowl stir together the sugar, vinegar, oil, garlic salt, pepper, and celery seed. Pour the dressing over the cabbage mixture; toss to coat.

Cover and chill at least 6 hours, stirring occasionally. Store, covered, in the refrigerator for up to 1 week. Use a slotted spoon to serve.

CORN BREAD SALAD

2 cups crumbled leftover corn bread—fat-free, of course
2 medium tomatoes, chopped
½ cup chopped scallions, tops and all
1 medium bell pepper, chopped
1 teaspoon seasoned salt
Dash of pepper
1 tablespoon sugar or Fructose
½ to ¾ cup fat-free mayonnaise (such as Miracle Whip)

SERVES 6

0 GRAMS FAT

Prep :15
Cook :00
Stand 1:00
Total 1:15

In a mixing bowl, combine the corn bread, tomatoes, scallions, and bell pepper.

In a separate small bowl, mix the seasoned salt, pepper, and sugar with the mayonnaise. Pour this dressing over the corn bread mixture and toss to combine. Let stand about 1 hour before serving.

MAKE-AHEAD MARINATED COLESLAW

SERVES 4

0 GRAMS FAT

Prep :15
Cook :04
Stand 8:00
Total 8:19

4 to 5 cups shredded cabbage (see Note)
1 medium onion, sliced thin
¾ cup sugar
¾ cup white vinegar
½ cup water
1 teaspoon celery seed
½ teaspoon dry mustard
½ teaspoon lemon pepper

Mix the cabbage and onion together in a large bowl with a lid that will seal, such as a Tupperware container.

In a saucepan, combine the remaining ingredients and boil for 3 to 4 minutes. Pour the hot dressing over the cabbage and onion and mix well. Cover and refrigerate for at least 8 hours, stirring two or three times. Use a slotted spoon for serving.

> *Note:* I use an old-fashioned kraut cutter to process my cabbage and onion, because when I make this it is usually for our church bean dinners and I make about three or four times this amount, so it takes a lot more shredding. It works great, but you need the kind with the sliding box on the top. This should keep some of you wondering. Check them out in the antique shops.

CRANBERRY SALAD

4 cups cranberries
1 cup sugar
1 (3-ounce) package red gelatin dessert mix
1 cup boiling water
1 cup cold water
¾ cup orange juice
1 (6-ounce) can crushed pineapple, drained
1 medium apple (not peeled), grated
½ cup finely chopped nuts (optional)

SERVES 6

0 GRAMS FAT IF NUTS OMITTED

Prep :25
Cook :00
Stand 4:00
Total 4:25

In a grinder or food processor, grind the cranberries. Transfer them to a medium-size bowl, add the sugar, and let stand until the sugar is dissolved.

Mix the gelatin with the hot and cold water and the orange juice. Let cool. Mix in the cranberries and add the drained pineapple and grated apple. Add nuts if using.

Stir, pour into your favorite mold or dish, and chill until firm.

Tip: Lovely for the holidays molded and set on a bed of shredded lettuce with green grapes arranged around the dish.

WARM GERMAN POTATO SALAD

SERVES 8

4 GRAMS FAT PER SERVING

Prep :10
Cook :20
Stand: 00
Total :30

10 cups cubed potatoes (about 3 pounds), peeled if desired (¼-inch cubes)
¾ cup chopped onion
1 (4-ounce) jar pimentos, drained and chopped
4 slices bacon

Dressing:
1 cup fat-free chicken broth
¾ cup vinegar
2 tablespoons canola oil
2 tablespoons flour
2 tablespoons sugar
½ teaspoon salt
½ teaspoon celery seed
¼ teaspoon pepper

Cover the potatoes with water and boil until tender, about 12 to 15 minutes. Drain and place in a large bowl. Add the onion and pimentos.

Meanwhile, in a large nonstick skillet, cook the bacon until crisp (I cook it in the microwave on a paper towel so it's less greasy). If using a regular skillet, when the bacon is crispy, remove and pat with a paper towel. Discard the bacon fat and wipe the skillet to remove any mean old grams hiding in there. Matter of fact, you'd better wash it with soap and water.

In the skillet, combine all the dressing ingredients. Whisk until blended and bring to a boil, whisking often. Reduce the heat and simmer 2 to 3 minutes, or until thickened. Pour over the potatoes and toss gently to coat. Crumble bacon over the top and serve immediately.

If you are being as careful as I had to be at first about the number of grams I consumed a day, you may desire to substitute bacon chips such as Baco or some such product for the bacon. Read your label to find the lowest in fat grams. You can still have the flavor without the 4 grams.

LIGHT AND ZESTY PASTA SALAD

½ cup fat-free Zesty Italian salad dressing
½ cup fat-free Miracle Whip salad dressing
1 cup broccoli florets
2 cups cooked corkscrew noodles, drained
½ cup chopped green pepper
½ cup chopped tomato
¼ cup sliced scallions

SERVES 4

LESS THAN 1
GRAM FAT PER
SERVING
(ONLY WHAT'S
IN PASTA)

Combine the dressings in a small bowl and mix well. Steam the broccoli just until crisp-tender. Drain and let cool.

In a large bowl, mix the broccoli florets with the pasta, green pepper, tomato, scallions, and dressing. Mix well. Chill 2 hours.

Prep :10
Cook :15
Stand 2:00
Total 2:25

GARDEN PASTA SALAD

SERVES 6

0 GRAMS FAT

Prep :15
Cook :14
Stand :00
Total :29

Dressing:
½ cup fat-free mayonnaise (such as Miracle Whip)
1 tablespoon vinegar
½ teaspoon Dijon mustard
½ teaspoon dried basil
½ teaspoon dried oregano
Dash ground red pepper
Dash black pepper

1 (16-ounce) package fettuccine, linguine, or spaghetti
½ pound broccoli florets
½ pound asparagus, cut into 1-inch pieces
1 (10-ounce) package frozen green peas, thawed and drained
1 green or red bell pepper, seeded and chopped coarse
½ pound mushrooms, sliced
¼ cup chopped parsley
½ cup grated fat-free Parmesan cheese

Prepare the salad dressing by placing all dressing ingredients in a jar and shaking well.

Prepare the pasta according to package directions, leaving out any oil or margarine called for; drain; place in a large bowl. Toss with about 1 tablespoon of the salad dressing. Set aside.

In a large saucepan, combine the broccoli and asparagus with boiling water to cover. Cook for about 4 minutes or until crisp-tender. Drain well and add to the pasta. Add the peas, bell pepper, mushrooms, parsley, and Parmesan. Toss thoroughly.

Pour remaining salad dressing over all and mix well.

RICE SALAD

3 cups cooked rice, chilled
¾ cup chopped scallions
½ cup chopped green pepper
½ cup chopped celery
½ cup chopped red bell pepper or pimento (adds color) (optional)

Dressing:
1 cup fat-free mayonnaise
1 tablespoon sugar or sweetener
1 teaspoon prepared mustard
Salt and pepper to taste
1 teaspoon vinegar

SERVES 6

TRACE OF FAT
PER 1-CUP
SERVING

Prep :15
Cook :00
Stand 2:00
Total 2:15

Mix the cold rice with the vegetables in a bowl.

In a separate bowl, combine the ingredients for the dressing. Pour the dressing over the rice mixture, and toss to combine thoroughly.

Chill at least 2 hours before serving. Garnish with tomato wedges if desired.

MANDARIN CHICKEN SALAD

A very pretty salad, especially for a ladies' luncheon or for your special friends.

SERVES 4

1 GRAM FAT PER SERVING

Prep :10
Cook :10
Stand :00
Total :20

1 (6-ounce) can mandarin orange segments, chilled
2 tablespoons rice vinegar or wine vinegar
⅓ cup honey
2 tablespoons reduced-sodium soy sauce
1 (8-ounce) can sliced water chestnuts, drained
4 cups shredded napa cabbage or lettuce
1 cup shredded red cabbage
½ cup thinly sliced radishes
4 slices red onion, cut in half and separated into half circles
4 boneless skinless chicken tenders, or any white meat pieces, cooked, cut into thin strips

Drain the oranges, reserving ⅓ cup of the liquid in a small mixing bowl. Into this reserved liquid, mix the vinegar, honey, and soy sauce. Blend with a wire whisk. Add the drained water chestnuts and set aside.

Divide the napa cabbage, red cabbage, radishes, and onion evenly onto four salad plates. Top with strips of chicken and orange segments. Remove the water chestnuts from the liquid with a slotted spoon and arrange on salads. Drizzle the remaining dressing over the salads.

CHICKEN WALDORF SALAD

2 cups cooked small shell pasta, cooled
1½ cups sliced celery
2 cups diced cooked or deli-style chicken breast
2 apples, peeled and diced
¼ cup sliced scallions
½ cup chopped and toasted walnuts

Dressing:
½ cup fat-free ranch dressing
3 tablespoons fat-free mayonnaise
1 tablespoon sugar
1 tablespoon cider vinegar
Dash of pepper
Lettuce leaves

Optional garnishes: avocado or mandarin orange slices

SERVES 4

3 GRAMS FAT
PER SERVING

Prep :15
Cook :10
Stand :30
Total :55

    In a large bowl, combine the pasta, celery, chicken, apples, scallions, and toasted walnuts.

    Prepare the dressing. In a small mixing bowl, combine the ranch dressing with the mayonnaise, sugar, vinegar, and pepper. Blend well and let stand at least 30 minutes, then add to the pasta mixture, tossing to coat thoroughly. To serve, mound on lettuce leaves. A slice of avocado or a few mandarin orange slices on the side are very pretty.

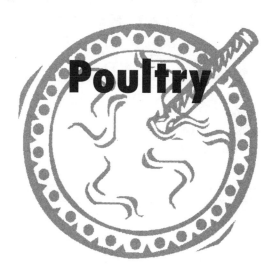

Poultry

CHICKEN WITH STUFFING—
SHORTCUT METHOD

SERVES 4

4 GRAMS FAT
PER SERVING

Prep :20
Cook 1:05
Stand :00
Total 1:25

1 (14-ounce) can fat-free chicken broth
2 tablespoons Butter Buds, liquid form
¾ cup chopped celery
¾ cup chopped onions
5 cups herb-seasoned or chicken-flavored packaged stuffing mix
4 boneless skinless chicken breast halves
2 tablespoons honey
2 tablespoons lemon juice
1 teaspoon parsley flakes

Preheat the oven to 375 degrees.

In a saucepan, combine the broth, Butter Buds, celery, and onions. Heat to boiling; simmer for 5 minutes or until the vegetables are crisp-tender. Remove from heat. Add stuffing mix and toss to combine.

Spray a 3-quart oblong baking dish with vegetable oil cooking spray. Spoon the stuffing mix into the dish and arrange the chicken down the center of the stuffing.

In a small bowl, combine the honey, lemon juice, and parsley flakes. Brush onto the chicken. Bake uncovered for 1 hour or until the chicken is tender. Stir the stuffing before serving.

VEGETABLE-STUFFED CHICKEN BREAST OVER RICE

4 boneless skinless chicken breast halves
2½ cups frozen veggies (broccoli, carrots, water chestnuts, red peppers)
½ cup fat-free chicken broth
¼ teaspoon thyme leaves
¼ teaspoon salt
¼ teaspoon paprika
⅛ teaspoon pepper
2 cups hot cooked rice (1 use Harvest Blend or wild or plain)
2 tablespoons flour
½ cup skim milk

SERVES 4

4 GRAMS FAT
PER SERVING

Prep :20
Cook :40
Stand :00
Total 1:00

Place a chicken breast half between two pieces of waxed paper or plastic wrap. Pound the chicken gently with a meat mallet or rolling pin until it is about ¼ inch thick. Repeat for the remaining chicken breasts.

Thaw the veggies by placing in a sieve and running hot water over them; shake any excess water off. Chop them fine and reserve about 1 cup for the sauce. Spoon some of the remaining veggies into the center of each chicken breast; roll up like a jelly roll.

In a large nonstick skillet, heat the chicken broth, thyme, salt, paprika, and pepper. Add the chicken rolls, seam side down. Bring to a boil, reduce the heat, cover, and simmer 20 to 25 minutes or until chicken is tender. Using a slotted spoon, remove chicken rolls. Arrange over cooked rice on a serving platter; cover to keep warm.

Add the reserved veggies to the mixture in the skillet. Bring to a boil, reduce the heat, and simmer for 5 to 6 minutes or until crisp-tender. In a small bowl, combine flour and milk, blend well, and add to the mixture in the skillet. Cook until thickened, stirring constantly. Spoon over the rice and chicken.

Serve with a nice garden salad.

BARBECUED CHICKEN

SERVES 4

4 GRAMS FAT PER SERVING

Prep :10
Cook :35
Stand :00
Total :45

4 skinless chicken breast halves, rib bone in
1 medium onion, cut into thin slices
1½ cups fat-free barbecue sauce (read label for 0 grams fat)

Preheat the oven to 350 degrees. Spray a 9 x 9-inch square baking dish lightly with vegetable oil cooking spray, or line it with foil. Set aside.

Wash the chicken breasts well and take off all visible fat. I use the bone-in chicken for barbecuing because it is moister than the breast without the bone. Cover the bottom of your baking dish with the onion. Place the chicken pieces bone side down in the baking dish and cover with foil. Bake for about 20 minutes. Uncover, drain off any juices collected in the baking dish, and spoon the barbecue sauce over the chicken generously. Return to the oven and continue to bake uncovered until tender. If you put the sauce on at the beginning it gets too saucy or dries out too much.

You can do this same recipe in a cooking bag for really easy cleanup, and it makes the chicken deliciously tender.

> *Variation:* You can cook these on your grill. First bake them in the oven for 20 minutes, covered, to make them nice and moist and tender. Then drain, coat with sauce, and place them bone side down on a hot grill until cooked through. This method takes a lot less grilling time and you can prepare them ahead of time and finish cooking when the guests arrive. Precooking also keeps them from getting dried out.

POT-ROASTED CHICKEN IN A BAG

No fuss—no muss. Throw away the mess of your stewpot.

SERVES 4

3.5 GRAMS FAT PER SERVING

Prep :15
Cook :50
Stand :00
Total 1:05

1 tablespoon flour
4 boneless skinless chicken breast halves
4 medium carrots, sliced
2 stalks celery, sliced
1 small whole onion, peeled
⅛ teaspoon garlic powder
½ cup brown gravy mix

Preheat the oven to 350 degrees. Place flour in a large (14 x 20-inch) oven bag; shake around to coat the inside of the bag. Place the bag in a 13 x 9-inch baking dish. Cut each chicken breast in half crosswise. Wash the chicken pieces and place in the bag along with the carrots, celery, and onion. Sprinkle garlic powder over all.

In a small bowl, combine the gravy mix with 1½ cups of water. Pour over the chicken and vegetables in the bag. Close the bag with a nylon tie. Cut 6 half-inch slits into the top of the bag to let steam escape.

Bake 45 to 50 minutes or until chicken is tender. Roll and move the bag around a couple of times during cooking to blend and coat all with gravy, being careful not to let it spill through the slits.

Variation: You can use lean pork in place of chicken, if desired.

BAG CHICKEN

SERVES 4

2.5 GRAMS FAT
PER SERVING

Prep :17
Cook 1:15
Stand :00
Total 1:32

1 tablespoon flour
4 to 6 boneless skinless chicken breast halves
½ cup chopped onion
½ cup chopped celery
1 cup whole-berry cranberry sauce
½ cup ketchup
1 tablespoon packed brown sugar
2 tablespoons lemon juice
1 tablespoon Worcestershire sauce
1 tablespoon prepared mustard
1 tablespoon red wine vinegar

Preheat the oven to 325 degrees. Place the flour in a large (14 x 20-inch) oven bag, shaking it to coat the inside. Put the bag in a 13 x 9 x 2-inch baking pan; set aside.

Dry-fry (in a nonstick skillet without any oil) the chicken breast until browned and tender. Remove with a slotted spoon and blot on paper towels to remove any oil that cooked out of the chicken.

Wipe out the skillet, add a tablespoon or two of water, and cook the onion and celery for 5 minutes, stirring often. Stir in the cranberry sauce and remaining ingredients. Bring to a slow boil. Place the chicken in the bag, spoon the sauce over the chicken, and close the bag as package directions suggest. Punch a few holes in top of the bag to let steam out.

Bake at 325 degrees for 1 hour and 15 minutes. About every 15 minutes, roll the bag around carefully to baste. (Be careful to keep the holes on top.) Serve with rice if desired.

OVEN "FRIED" CHICKEN

1/2 cup egg substitute
1 1/2 cups cornflake crumbs
4 boneless skinless chicken breast halves

SERVES 4

4 GRAMS FAT
PER SERVING

Prep :10
Cook :35
Stand :00
Total :45

Preheat the oven to 375 degrees. Lightly spray a baking sheet with vegetable oil cooking spray.

In two small shallow separate bowls, place the egg substitute and cornflake crumbs. One at a time, dip each piece of chicken into the egg substitute, then roll in the crumbs, patting to make sure they are coated well. This will make them nice and crispy. Place on the cooking sheet. Spray each piece lightly with vegetable oil cooking spray.

Bake for 30 to 35 minutes or until tender and crispy, turning each piece after 15 minutes.

CAJUN OVEN "FRIED" CHICKEN

1/2 cup egg substitute
1 1/2 cups corn flake crumbs
4 boneless skinless chicken breast halves
1/2 teaspoon crushed oregano leaves
1/4 teaspoon cayenne pepper
1/2 teaspoon garlic powder
2 tablespoons Creole seasoning

SERVES 4

4 GRAMS PER
SERVING

Prep :10
Cook :35
Stand :00
Total :45

Preheat the oven to 350 degrees. Lightly spray a baking sheet well with vegetable cooking spray; set aside.

Take two small shallow bowls and put the egg substitute in one and the corn flake crumbs in the other. Mix the seasonings with the corn flake crumbs, being sure they are mixed well.

Coat the chicken, one piece at a time, with the egg substitute, then roll in the corn flake crumbs, patting to make sure the pieces are coated well. This will make it nice and crispy. *(continued)*

Place on the prepared baking sheet and spray the top of each piece with vegetable cooking spray lightly. Bake for about 30 to 35 minutes, turning each piece when half done. You may want to vary the seasonings—it may be a little too hot for some.

CHICKEN BREASTS WITH SWEET ORANGE SAUCE

SERVES 8

3 GRAMS FAT
PER SERVING

Prep :15
Cook 1:00
Stand :00
Total 1:15

8 boneless skinless chicken breast halves
1½ cups herb-seasoned stuffing mix
¼ cup Butter Buds, liquid form
½ cup orange juice
4 cups hot cooked wild rice
Sweet Orange Sauce (see below)

Preheat the oven to 350 degrees. Lightly coat a 13 x 9-inch baking dish with vegetable oil cooking spray. Arrange the chicken breasts in the dish and sprinkle some of the stuffing mix over each. Drizzle with Butter Buds and then with the orange juice. Cover the dish tightly with foil and bake for 1 hour. Serve with wild rice and Sweet Orange Sauce.

Sweet Orange Sauce

1 (6-ounce) can frozen orange juice concentrate, thawed and undiluted
½ cup orange marmalade
2 tablespoons steak sauce

Combine all ingredients in a microwave-safe container. Microwave on high 6 minutes or until hot and bubbly, stirring once. Spoon over chicken on a bed of wild rice.

SPICY MEXICAN CHICKEN

½ cup fine dry bread crumbs
¼ cup fat-free Parmesan cheese
1 teaspoon chili powder
¼ teaspoon ground cumin
¼ teaspoon pepper
8 boneless skinless chicken breast halves
2 cups shredded fat-free Monterey Jack cheese
½ cup egg substitute

SERVES 8

4 GRAMS FAT
PER SERVING

Prep :10
Cook :40
Stand :00
Total :50

Preheat the oven to 375 degrees. Lightly coat an 11 x 7-inch baking dish with vegetable oil cooking spray.

In a shallow dish, combine the bread crumbs, Parmesan cheese, chili powder, cumin, and pepper. Set aside.

Place each chicken breast between two sheets of wax paper; flatten to a thickness of ¼ inch with a meat mallet or rolling pin. Place ¼ cup of shredded cheese in the middle of each piece of chicken, roll up from short side, and secure with a wooden pick. Dip the chicken rolls in the egg substitute and dredge in the bread crumb mixture. Place rolls seam side down in the prepared baking dish. Spray the pieces of chicken very lightly with vegetable oil cooking spray and bake for 35 to 40 minutes. Depending on the size of chicken pieces, cooking time may vary.

Variation: If you don't have time to flatten the chicken, just skip that step. Dip the chicken in the egg substitute, then dredge in bread crumbs, spray, and bake. About the last 5 minutes of baking time, put the shredded cheese on the top of each piece and melt. A little dollop of chopped green chiles on top of the cheese is also very good.

SERVES 4

**3 GRAMS FAT
PER SERVING**

**Prep :15
Cook :45
Stand :00
Total 1:00**

KRISPY CHICKEN

4 cups Rice Krispies
1 teaspoon paprika
½ teaspoon salt (optional)
¼ teaspoon pepper
4 boneless skinless chicken breast halves
¾ cup fat-free mayonnaise

Preheat the oven to 400 degrees. Spray a baking sheet lightly with vegetable oil cooking spray.

In a large zipper-lock plastic bag, place the Rice Krispies; close the bag and crush with a rolling pin. Add the paprika, salt, if desired, and pepper. Set aside.

Wash chicken pieces and pat dry. Cover each piece with mayonnaise and place, one at a time, in the bag of Rice Krispies. Shake to cover well. Place the chicken on the prepared baking sheet and bake for 40 to 45 minutes, until crisp and brown.

SERVES 4

**3 GRAMS FAT
PER SERVING**

**Prep :10
Cook :15
Stand 6:00
Total 6:25**

MIRACLE CHICKEN

4 boneless skinless chicken breast halves
¾ cup fat-free Miracle Whip salad dressing
1 cup fat-free Italian salad dressing
¼ cup dry white wine

Place the chicken breast halves in one layer in a baking dish or deep platter.

Stir together the Miracle Whip, Italian dressing, and wine. Pour this marinade over the chicken pieces. Cover and refrigerate for several hours or overnight.

Preheat a gas grill or an oven broiler, or start a charcoal fire. Spray the grill or broiler rack lightly with vegetable oil cooking spray before lighting the fire.

Drain the chicken, reserving the marinade, and arrange on the grill. Cook about 5 to 7 minutes on each side, brushing frequently with the reserved marinade. Discard the remaining marinade.

CHICKEN WITH BROCCOLI AND RICE CASSEROLE

4 boneless skinless chicken breast halves
Garlic powder and pepper
1 (10 ¾-ounce) can Healthy Request cream of broccoli soup
½ soup can water (swish water around to get all the soup)
4 cups cooked rice or pasta

SERVES 4

4.25 GRAMS FAT PER SERV- ING

Prep :10
Cook 1:00
Stand :00
Total 1:10

Preheat the oven to 375 degrees.

Lightly spray a 2-quart cooking dish with vegetable oil cooking spray; arrange the chicken in a single layer in the dish. Sprinkle with garlic powder and pepper to taste.

Bake for about 30 minutes. Drain off any juices (they will contain some fat that has cooked out of the chicken).

Combine the soup and water and mix with a wire whisk. Pour over the chicken and bake an additional 30 minutes or until the chicken is done.

Serve with rice cooked according to package directions.

CHICKEN AND PASTA SKILLET DINNER

SERVES 4

1.5 GRAMS FAT PER 2-CUP SERVING

Prep :10
Cook :35
Stand :00
Total :45

1½ cups pasta (I use ziti or any large tubular pasta)
6 frozen breaded chicken tenders
½ cup chopped onions
¾ cup chopped celery
½ cup chopped green peppers
1 (14-ounce) can stewed tomatoes
½ tomato can water (about ¾ cup)
½ teaspoon crushed dried basil
½ teaspoon lemon pepper
½ teaspoon crushed dried oregano
¼ teaspoon pizza (mild Italian) seasoning
2 cups chopped raw cabbage
1 cup frozen green peas

In a medium saucepan, cook the pasta according to package directions, leaving out salt and oil if called for. Drain. Set aside.

While the pasta is cooking, start your dish. In a large or deep nonstick skillet or dutch oven, brown the chicken tenders lightly.

Add the chopped onions, celery, and peppers; sauté until just starting to soften. Cut the chicken into bite-size pieces with a spatula. Add the stewed tomatoes, water, basil, lemon pepper, oregano leaves, and pizza seasoning. Simmer for about 5 minutes; add the cabbage and green peas. Continue simmering, stirring occasionally, until vegetables are desired tenderness.

Carefully stir in the pasta and simmer a few minutes longer. Add a little more water if the mixture seems too thick or dry.

CHICKEN BROCCOLI BAKE

2 cups chopped broccoli florets
2 cups diced cooked chicken (white meat)
1 (10¾-ounce) can Healthy Request low-fat cream of mushroom soup
1 cup fat-free mayonnaise
1 teaspoon lemon juice
1½ cups shredded fat-free Cheddar cheese

SERVES 6

3 GRAMS FAT
PER 1½-CUP
SERVING

Prep :20
Cook :35
Stand :00
Total :55

Preheat the oven to 350 degrees. Lightly spray a 9 x 13-inch baking dish with vegetable oil cooking spray.

Steam the broccoli just until crisp-tender. Drain. Layer the broccoli in the prepared baking dish. Layer the chicken on top of the broccoli.

In a mixing bowl, combine the soup, mayonnaise, and lemon juice. Spread evenly over the chicken. Top with cheese. Bake uncovered for 30 minutes, or until bubbly.

LADIES' LUNCHEON CASSEROLE

I buy frozen diced chicken at a wholesale store to have on hand at all times for just this kind of a recipe, which you can throw together in a hurry and look like you have been working for hours. I'll never tell if you don't.

2 cups diced cooked chicken (white meat)
2 cups cooked rice
1 (10¾-ounce) can Healthy Request cream of mushroom soup
1 (10¾-ounce) can Healthy Request cream of broccoli soup
1 (8-ounce) can sliced water chestnuts, drained
1 (11-ounce) can white shoepeg corn, drained
Salt and pepper to taste

SERVES 6

1 GRAM FAT
PER 1½-CUP
SERVING

Prep :10
Cook :45
Stand :00
Total :55

Preheat the oven to 350 degrees. Lightly spray a 2-quart baking dish with vegetable oil cooking spray.   *(continued)*

In a large bowl, combine the cooked chicken with the rice and cream of mushroom soup. Fill the soup can ½ full of water, swish it around to loosen any soup left behind, and add to above. Repeat with the cream of broccoli soup. Add the water chestnuts, corn, and salt and pepper to taste. Stir to blend all ingredients.

Spoon into the prepared baking dish and bake uncovered for about 45 minutes, until bubbly and heated through.

CHICKEN CASSEROLE

SERVES 8

3 GRAMS FAT PER SERVING

Prep :20
Cook 1:00
Stand :00
Total 1:20

10 slices low-fat (1 gram per slice) white bread, cut into 1-inch cubes
1½ cups fat-free cracker crumbs
3 cups fat-free chicken broth
¾ cup egg substitute, lightly beaten
¾ cup diced celery
3 tablespoons chopped onion
3 cups cubed cooked chicken breast
1 (8-ounce) can sliced mushrooms, drained
1 cup whole-kernel corn (optional)
Salt to taste (about 1 teaspoon)

Preheat the oven to 350 degrees. Lightly coat a 2-quart casserole with butter-flavored vegetable oil cooking spray.

In a large mixing bowl, combine the bread cubes and 1 cup of the cracker crumbs. Stir in the chicken broth, egg substitute, celery, onion, chicken, and mushrooms. Add corn if desired and salt to taste. Spoon into the prepared casserole.

In a nonstick skillet, place the remaining ½ cup of cracker crumbs. Spray with butter-flavored cooking spray, stirring to coat evenly. Cook, stirring, until lightly browned. Sprinkle over the casserole. Bake uncovered for 1 hour.

Note: You may make this a day ahead. Leave off the top cracker crumbs until time for baking.

CHICKEN, VEGETABLES, AND DUMPLINGS

6 boneless skinless chicken breast halves
½ cup chopped onion
1 cup chopped celery
1 cup chopped carrots
2 cups skim milk

Dumplings:
1½ cups self-rising flour
¾ cup skim milk
2 tablespoons cornstarch
Salt and pepper to taste

SERVES 6

3 GRAMS FAT
PER 1-CUP
SERVING

Prep :35
Cook :45
Stand :00
Total 1:20

Wash the chicken and trim off any visible fat. In a large saucepan, cover the chicken with water, bring to a boil, and lower the heat to medium. Add the onion, celery, and carrots; cook 25 minutes or until tender.

Strain through a colander, reserving broth and solids separately.

Defat the broth with a defatting pitcher or dipper, or if none is available, cool the broth and place in the refrigerator overnight or for a few hours and remove any excess fat, which will come to the top.

About a half hour before you want to serve, return the chicken and vegetables to the defatted broth. Add 2 cups of skim milk and bring all to a boil. While the chicken and vegetables are heating, prepare the dumplings.

Dumplings: In a mixing bowl, combine the self-rising flour with ¾ cup of milk. Stir the milk in gradually, ¼ cup at a time. Mix with a fork until a soft dough forms.

Drop the dumplings by the tablespoonful into the boiling liquid. Let boil without stirring for 15 minutes. Do not cover.

In a small bowl, combine the cornstarch and 2 tablespoons *cold* water. Turn heat off, carefully stir this into the chicken and dumpling broth—not too vigorously or you'll mush up the dumplings and vegetables. Add salt and pepper to taste. *(continued)*

Serve directly from the pot or transfer to a platter and pass the sauce separately.

> *Variation:* Chicken Potpie: You may roll the dough out thin on a floured surface, adding enough flour to make the dough workable. Cut into 1½-inch squares with a sharp knife. If you like tender potpie dumplings, cook immediately. If you like tougher dumplings like Grandma used to make, let them sit for about 1 hour after you roll them out and cut them. You may not need to thicken the broth, as the excess flour will probably make it thick enough. If not, then use the cornstarch.

BUSY DAY CROCK-POT CHICKEN SPECIAL

This is for the working person who savors the flavor as well as their time.

SERVES 4

3 GRAMS FAT PER SERVING

Prep :12
Cook 6:00
Stand :00
Total 6:12

4 boneless skinless chicken breast halves
1 (10-ounce) package frozen mixed vegetables (mixture of diced carrots, green beans, etc.)
1 medium onion, cut into thick slices or chunks
¾ to 1 cup sliced fresh mushrooms
1 (14-ounce) can stewed tomatoes
1 (8-ounce) can tomato sauce
1 teaspoon dried Italian seasoning, crushed
2 cloves garlic, minced

Cut the chicken into 1-inch pieces. Place the mixed vegetables, onion, and mushrooms in a Crock-Pot (about 4 quarts or larger). Place the chicken pieces on top of the vegetables.

In a medium-size mixing bowl, combine the tomatoes with their juice, the tomato sauce, Italian seasoning, and garlic. Pour over the chicken and vegetables.

Cover and cook for 6 hours on low heat setting or 3 hours on high.

Serve this over hot rice or fettuccine, cooked and drained, along with garlic bread or toast. (Spray bread slices with vegetable oil cooking spray and sprinkle with garlic salt. Toast on both sides in a nonstick skillet or grill until golden.)

STIR-FRY CHICKEN AND VEGGIES

3 boneless skinless chicken breast halves
¼ cup low-sodium soy sauce
1 teaspoon sesame seeds
1 medium onion, chopped
1 medium green pepper, chopped
4 cups frozen stir-fry vegetables
1 (4-ounce) can mushroom pieces, drained
1 (4-ounce) can sliced water chestnuts, drained

SERVES 4

2 GRAMS FAT
ENTIRE DISH

Prep :15
Cook :10
Stand :00
Total :25

Cut the chicken breast into 1-inch squares. In a nonstick skillet or wok, brown the chicken pieces until light brown. Add the soy sauce and sesame seeds; continue to cook until tender. With a slotted spoon remove the chicken to a platter; set aside.

To the juices in the same pan, add the onions and green pepper; cook until crisp-tender. Add the frozen vegetables, mushroom pieces, and water chestnuts. Cook, stirring constantly, until all is hot. Return the chicken to the vegetable mixture and stir in. Serve with hot rice if desired.

CHICKEN VEGETABLE SPECIAL

I use a large electric nonstick skillet for this and serve it with a pone of cornbread alongside a small green salad.

SERVES 4

**3.0 GRAMS FAT
ENTIRE DISH**

**Prep :25
Cook :30
Stand :00
Total :55**

6 frozen chicken tenders
¾ cup uncooked flat noodles
1½ cups okra
1½ cups chopped cabbage
1 tablespoon vinegar
⅔ cup chopped onion
⅔ cup chopped green pepper
1 cup chopped celery
1 (14-ounce) can stewed tomatoes, pasta style
¾ cup picante sauce (commercial)
½ teaspoon minced garlic
½ teaspoon crushed oregano leaves
½ teaspoon crushed dried basil
¼ teaspoon Creole seasoning
¼ teaspoon adobo seasoning
½ teaspoon lemon pepper

In a nonstick skillet, dry-fry the chicken tenders until brown. In a medium saucepan, cook the noodles according to package directions, leaving out any oil or margarine called for. (Salt may also be omitted.)

If using fresh okra, trim the ends, slice ½ inch thick, and cover with water in a saucepan. Add about 1 tablespoon vinegar and boil 4 to 5 minutes, until crisp-tender. Drain in a colander and rinse with warm water.

Cut the chicken into bite-size pieces, return to the skillet, and add the onions, green pepper, and celery. Sauté until slightly tender (add ¼ cup water if needed).

Add the tomatoes and ½ can of water, the picante sauce, and seasonings. Simmer for about 5 minutes. Add the noodles, okra, and cabbage; continue to simmer about 5 more minutes—the cabbage should be crisp-tender. Be careful when stirring not to break up the noodles too much.

BAYOU MAGIC CHICKEN

4 to 6 frozen chicken tenders
¾ cup chopped onion
3⅓ cups chopped celery
1 small green pepper, chopped
1 (10¾-ounce) can Healthy Request cream of mushroom soup
1 (10¾-ounce) can Healthy Request cream of celery soup
1 (16-ounce) can Healthy Request (or fat-free) chicken broth
1 (14-ounce) package Bayou Magic Cajun rice mix

SERVES 8

3 GRAMS FAT
PER SERVING

Prep :10
Cook 1:40
Stand :00
Total 1:50

Put the chicken tenders, onion, celery, and pepper in a nonstick skillet over medium heat. When they start to brown, add 1 cup water. Simmer 20 minutes, or until tender and thick. Cut the chicken tenders into bite-size pieces.

Add the mushroom and celery soups, 2 soup cans of water, and the chicken broth. While this is heating a little, put the rice into a colander or strainer and shake some of the pepper out (it is seasoned too hot for us Okies; if you are in Cajun country, then just leave all spices in). Add the rice to the above mixture. Place in a casserole about 11 x 13 inches, cover with foil, and bake at 350 degrees for 1 hour and 10 minutes or until the rice is tender.

QUICK SPICY CHICKEN GUMBO

Be creative in the summer when the fresh vegetables are plentiful. Add all your favorites.

SERVES 4

3.0 GRAMS FAT
ENTIRE DISH

Prep :10
Cook :20
Stand :00
Total :30

1 cup sliced fresh or frozen okra (optional)
1 teaspoon vinegar
6 boneless skinless chicken tenders
½ pound fat-free smoked sausage such as Butterball, cut into ½-inch slices
½ cup chopped onion
½ cup chopped green peppers
½ teaspoon chopped garlic
1 (16-ounce) package frozen vegetables, such as broccoli, corn, peppers, etc.
1 (14-ounce) can stewed tomatoes
Salt and pepper

If using okra, cover it with water in a saucepan, add 1 teaspoon of vinegar, and boil 4 or 5 minutes, or until just tender. Rinse in a colander. (This process will eliminate any slimy texture in your gumbo.) Set aside.

In a large deep nonstick skillet, cook the chicken tenders and sausage pieces until tender and lightly browned. Remove from the skillet and cut the chicken into ½-inch chunks.

In the same skillet, sauté the onion, peppers, and garlic in ¼ cup of water for 5 minutes. Return the chicken and sausage to the skillet and add the frozen vegetables, the okra, the tomatoes, and 1 cup of water. Cover and cook over medium heat about 3 to 5 minutes. Season with salt and pepper; serve hot.

QUICK CHICKEN GUMBO

1½ to 2 cups frozen fully cooked hickory-flavored chicken, thawed and cut into
    bite-size pieces (or cubed uncooked white meat chicken)
¼ cup chopped green peppers
1 (12-ounce) package frozen gumbo mix
1 (8-ounce) can stewed tomatoes
½ teaspoon garlic flakes
1 cup cooked macaroni

SERVES 2

2 GRAMS FAT
PER SERVING

Prep :08
Cook :25
Stand :00
Total :33

In a nonstick skillet, cook the chicken in ¼ cup water along with
the peppers until tender.

In a separate saucepan cover the gumbo mix with ¼ cup of water
and simmer for 4 to 5 minutes. Drain in a colander and add to the
chicken in the skillet along with the tomatoes and garlic flakes.
Simmer for 15 to 20 minutes. Add cooked macaroni; stir in gently
to avoid breaking.

Variation: A touch of Cajun seasoning may be added to your
taste. Omit the macaroni and serve on rice.

CREOLE CHICKEN AND PASTA

6 fresh or frozen chicken tenders
¾ cup chopped onion
¾ cup chopped green pepper
1 (12-ounce) package frozen gumbo mix
1 tablespoon vinegar
2 cups uncooked ziti
1½ cups tomato juice
½ cup fat-free spaghetti sauce
½ teaspoon crushed dried basil
½ teaspoon crushed dried oregano
Dash lemon pepper
Dash adobo seasoning

SERVES 6

1 GRAM FAT
PER 1½-CUP
SERVING

Prep :15
Cook :50
Stand :00
Total 1:05

Dry-fry the chicken tenders in a nonstick skillet. Add the onion and green pepper when the chicken is about ¾ of the way done and lightly browned. Take the chicken out of the skillet (so as not to scratch the skillet), cut it into bite-size pieces, and return to the skillet.

While the chicken is cooking, in a separate saucepan cook the vegetable gumbo mix according to package directions. Add a tablespoon of vinegar to keep the okra from being slick. Drain in a colander when tender. Set aside.

Cook the pasta until tender in a separate pan; drain and set aside.

To the chicken and vegetables in the skillet, add the tomato juice and spaghetti sauce and stir in ¾ cup of water. Bring to a boil and add the seasonings, the reserved gumbo mix, and the pasta. Stir carefully, lower the heat, and simmer for about 20 minutes, until the flavors are blended.

CHICKEN CHILI

The corn gives this and other chilies, soups, and chowders a wonderful crunch.

SERVES 4

6 GRAMS FAT
PER 1¼-CUP
SERVING

Prep :20
Cook :30
Stand :00
Total :50

2 cups ground chicken or turkey (use freshly ground for less fat)
1 cup chopped onion
¾ cup chopped green pepper
1 cup chopped carrot
2 Roma or other small tomatoes, chopped
4 rings jalapeño pepper, chopped fine
1 (15-ounce) can Great Northern beans, drained
1 (11-ounce) can white shoepeg corn, drained
2 (14-ounce) cans fat-free chicken broth
2 teaspoons chili powder, or more to taste
½ teaspoon ground cumin

In a large nonstick skillet or saucepan, brown the chicken, onion, and green pepper over medium heat, stirring often. Transfer to a colander and run hot water over to rinse away any excess fat. Shake to remove water and return to the skillet after wiping out any fat. Add the carrots and remaining ingredients, bring to a boil, reduce the heat, cover, and simmer for 15 minutes.

HURRY-SCURRY CHICKEN CHILI

4 frozen chicken tenders
½ cup chopped onions
1½ cups Harvest Blend rice
1 (14-ounce) can fat-free vegetable chili
2 (12-ounce) cans chili beans
1 tablespoon chili powder
Dash of adobo seasoning

SERVES 2

4 GRAMS FAT
PER 2½-CUP
SERVING

Prep :20
Cook :15
Stand :00
Total :35

In a nonstick skillet, dry-fry the chicken tenders and onions 5 to 8 minutes, or until tender. You may add about 2 tablespoons of water to speed up and tenderize. Cut into bite-size pieces (I use the rubber or plastic spatula).

In a small saucepan, cook the rice according to package directions, leaving out the margarine or butter.

In a large heavy saucepan, pour the chili right from the can, as well as the two cans of beans. Add the rice and chicken. Stir in the seasonings and simmer for 15 to 20 minutes.

BAKED CHICKEN CHILI CASSEROLE

SERVES 4

4 GRAMS FAT
PER SERVING

Prep :15
Cook 1:10
Stand :00
Total 1:25

½ cup uncooked Harvest Blend rice
1 (14-ounce) can fat-free chicken broth
2 cups chopped cooked chicken breast
1½ cups medium salsa
1 (10¾-ounce) can Healthy Request cream of chicken soup
1 cup whole-kernel corn, frozen or canned, drained
½ cup finely chopped onion
1 tablespoon lite Worcestershire sauce
2 tablespoons chili powder, or to taste
1 teaspoon dried oregano
¼ teaspoon pepper

Preheat the oven to 350 degrees. Lightly coat a 2-quart baking dish with vegetable oil cooking spray.

In a saucepan, combine the rice and chicken broth; bring to a boil. Cover, reduce the heat, and simmer 40 minutes or until rice is tender.

Combine the chicken and remaining ingredients in a large bowl; stir in the rice. Spoon the mixture into the prepared baking dish and bake for 30 minutes or until bubbly.

TORTILLA CASSEROLE

2 pounds ground turkey
1 cup chopped onion
1 clove garlic, minced
1 (15-ounce) can tomato sauce
1 (2-ounce) package taco seasoning
1 (4-ounce) can green chiles
1 teaspoon chili powder, or more to taste
Salt and pepper to taste (optional)
12 (6-inch) corn tortillas
1 (10¾-ounce) can Healthy Request low-fat cream of chicken soup
¾ cup skim milk
2 cups shredded fat-free cheddar cheese

SERVES 6

2 GRAMS FAT
PER SERVING

Prep :20
Cook 1:10
Stand :00
Total 1:30

Preheat the oven to 350 degrees.

Brown the turkey, onion, and garlic in a nonstick skillet over medium heat, stirring frequently. Transfer to a colander, rinse under hot water to remove any fat, and shake excess water off. With a paper towel, remove any fat in the skillet. Return the turkey to the skillet; add the tomato sauce, taco seasoning, green chiles, chili powder, and salt and pepper if desired. Mix well and heat thoroughly.

Line a 9 x 13-inch baking dish with half the tortillas. Spoon the turkey mixture over the tortillas. Layer the remaining tortillas over the turkey mixture and pour the soup over the tortillas. Pour the milk over the soup. Sprinkle cheese over all and bake uncovered for 45 minutes. Serve with salsa and fat-free sour cream if desired.

CHICKEN ENCHILADAS

SERVES 6

4.34 GRAMS FAT PER SERVING

Prep :40
Cook 1:05
Stand :00
Total 1:45

5 boneless skinless chicken breast halves
2 (3-ounce) packages fat-free cream cheese, at room temperature
⅓ cup evaporated skim milk
¾ cup chopped onion
½ teaspoon salt (optional)
2 cups tomatillo sauce
12 (6-inch) corn tortillas
1 cup shredded fat-free Cheddar cheese
1 cup shredded fat-free Monterey Jack cheese

In a large saucepan, cover the chicken with water, bring to a boil, reduce the heat, and simmer about 40 minutes, or until tender. Remove the chicken and, when cool enough to handle, chop fine.

Preheat the oven to 350 degrees. Spray a 9 x 13-inch baking dish lightly with vegetable oil cooking spray.

Combine the softened cream cheese and the milk in a mixing bowl and whisk together until smooth. Stir in the chicken, onion, and salt, if desired. Set aside.

Spread ¾ cup tomatillo sauce in the prepared baking dish.

Soften the tortillas by dipping each, one at a time, in a shallow dish of warm water briefly, or wrap the stack in foil and warm in oven ahead of time.

Spoon about 1½ tablespoons tomatillo sauce over each tortilla, spreading to the edge; spoon ¼ cup of the chicken mixture evenly down center of each. Roll up the tortillas and place seam side down in the baking dish.

Cover with foil and bake the enchiladas for about 25 minutes. Uncover, sprinkle with cheeses, and return to the oven long enough to melt the cheese. Serve garnished with fat-free sour cream.

SWEET-AND-SOUR CHICKEN AND RICE

1 (8-ounce) bottle fat-free French dressing
1 (8-ounce) jar apricot preserves
½ cup honey
1 envelope Lipton onion soup mix
6 boneless skinless chicken tenders
1 cup rice, prepared according to package directions, leaving out the butter or
    margarine and salt

In a medium-size mixing bowl, combine the French dressing, preserves, honey, and soup mix. Set the sauce aside.

In a nonstick skillet, dry-fry the chicken tenders until done. Add the sauce, simmer for about 5 minutes, and stir in the rice, if desired; or the chicken and sauce may be served on top of the rice.

SERVES 4

1.25 GRAMS
FAT PER SERV-
ING

Prep :10
Cook :20
Stand :00
Total :30

CHICKEN CHILES CASSEROLE

Cooked turkey or ham may be substituted for the chicken in this easy day-ahead dish. Prepare, cover, and refrigerate until ready to bake.

1 cup fat-free sour cream
1 cup Healthy Request cream of chicken soup
1 cup chopped onion
1 (4-ounce) can chopped green chiles
½ cup chopped green pepper
1 teaspoon salt
½ teaspoon pepper
1 (2-pound) package frozen hash brown potatoes, with peppers and onions
2½ cups chopped cooked white meat chicken
2½ cups shredded fat-free Cheddar cheese

SERVES 6

1 GRAM FAT
PER 1-CUP
SERVING

Prep :10
Cook 1:15
Stand :00
Total 1:25

Preheat the oven to 350 degrees. Lightly coat a 13 x 9-inch baking dish with vegetable oil cooking spray.

In a large bowl, mix the sour cream, soup, onion, chiles, green pepper, salt, and pepper. Stir in the potatoes, chicken, and 2 cups of the cheese. Pour into the prepared baking dish. Bake uncovered for 1 hour and 15 minutes or until golden brown. Sprinkle with the remaining cheese before serving.

GRILLED CHICKEN CHEESE SANDWICH

Quick, easy, and good. Serve with chips and salsa if desired.

SERVES 4

2 GRAMS FAT
PER SERVING

Prep :10
Cook :08
Stand :00
Total :18

8 slices low-fat bread (1 gram per slice)
4 teaspoons fat-free sandwich spread (such as Miracle Whip)
4 slices fat-free deli-style chicken (such as Healthy Choice)
2 thin slices onion separated into rings
4 tablespoons salsa
4 slices fat-free Cheddar or American cheese

Heat a nonstick skillet or a grill over medium heat. Spread each slice of bread with sandwich spread. On four of the slices layer a slice of chicken, some onion rings, 1 tablespoon of salsa, and a slice of cheese. Top with the remaining slices of bread.

Spray the skillet lightly with vegetable oil cooking spray, place the sandwiches in the skillet, and spray the top of each lightly with cooking spray. When lightly browned, turn over with a spatula. Brown lightly on the other side. Transfer to a platter and cut in half diagonally.

CHICKEN CHEESEBURGERS

These taste great! Your craving for a burger has been taken care of and so has your fat gram count.

4 boneless skinless chicken breast halves
4 slices fat-free Cheddar cheese
4 light hamburger buns
Lettuce, onion, pickles, tomatoes, mustard

SERVES 4

5 GRAMS FAT
PER SERVING

Prep :10
Cook :15
Stand :00
Total :25

Remove any fat from chicken breast. Grill on a preheated outdoor grill or cook in a nonstick skillet, turning once, for about 5 minutes per side, until just cooked through.

Carefully, so as not to burn your fingers, split the chicken pieces almost through, butterfly fashion. Open and lay them flat on the grill or in the skillet. Place a slice of cheese on top and cook only until the cheese is melted. You don't want to dry out the chicken.

Meanwhile, while the cheese is melting, open the buns and place on the grill or around the chicken in the skillet. When all is hot and melted, place each opened bun on a serving plate and top with a piece of chicken. Add all the trimmings as you would a regular hamburger.

ZITI TURKEY CASSEROLE

SERVES 8

2 GRAMS FAT
PER SERVING

Prep :35
Cook 1:20
Stand :15
Total 2:10

This is a great do-ahead dish for entertaining or for family-night supper at church. You can use lean beef instead of turkey, although it will add more fat grams.

2 cups chopped onions
1½ pounds lean ground turkey
1 (8-ounce) can tomato sauce
¼ cup chopped fresh parsley
½ teaspoon dried oregano
½ teaspoon salt
½ teaspoon pepper
1 pound ziti (or other tubular pasta), prepared according to package directions
     (about 10 cups)

Sauce:
1 (8-ounce) can tomato sauce
Pinch of oregano
Pinch of dried basil
1 cup fat-free Parmesan cheese

Preheat the oven to 350 degrees. Lightly spray a deep 3-quart casserole with vegetable oil cooking spray.

In a large nonstick skillet, dry-fry the onions, adding about 2 tablespoons water if needed, for 5 to 6 minutes, or until translucent. Add the turkey, stirring to break up lumps, and cook 8 to 10 minutes or until lightly browned. Transfer to a colander; rinse with hot water to remove any excess fat. Wipe the skillet clean of any fat with paper towels.

Return the meat to the skillet; add ¼ cup water, the can of tomato sauce, and the parsley, oregano, salt, and pepper. Simmer over medium heat 2 to 3 minutes or until the liquid is almost gone. Remove from heat.

Spread half of the cooked, drained ziti evenly in the prepared casserole. Spread the meat mixture over the pasta. Top with the remaining ziti.

In a small mixing bowl, mix the remaining can of tomato sauce with a pinch each of oregano and basil and half the Parmesan cheese. Pour over the casserole; top with the remaining Parmesan. Bake uncovered for 1 hour, or until lightly browned. Let stand 15 minutes before serving.

> *Note:* You can make this ahead. After assembling, refrigerate uncovered until cool, then cover with plastic wrap and refrigerate up to 3 days. If made ahead, allow to stand at room temperature for 20 minutes before putting in the oven. Bake 1 hour and 15 minutes. Let stand 15 minutes before serving.

SOUTH OF THE BORDER CASSEROLE

8 or 9 (6-inch) corn tortillas
½ pound lean (93% fat-free) fresh ground turkey
¾ cup chopped onion
1 cup mild or medium taco sauce
1 (4-ounce) can chopped green chiles
¾ cup frozen whole-kernel corn, thawed
¾ cup shredded fat-free Cheddar cheese
Fat-free sour cream, if desired for garnish
2 green onions, chopped, if desired for garnish

SERVES 4

6 GRAMS FAT
PER SERVING

Prep :15
Cook :35
Stand :00
Total :50

Preheat the oven to 350 degrees. Lightly coat a 1½-quart casserole with vegetable oil cooking spray.

Place the tortillas on a cookie sheet, not overlapping, and bake until crisp, about 4 minutes on one side; turn and bake 2 more minutes on the other. Cool on a wire rack. (Leave the oven on.)

In a nonstick skillet, dry-fry the turkey and onion, stirring to break up lumps, until the turkey is brown. Transfer to a colander and rinse off any fat with hot water. Shake to remove water. Wipe the skillet with paper towels to remove any fat that cooked out of the turkey. Return the turkey and onion to the skillet; add the taco sauce, chiles, and corn. Bring to a boil, reduce the heat, and simmer for about 5 minutes.

Break up 3 of the tortillas and arrange over the bottom of the prepared casserole.

Spoon half the turkey mixture over the tortillas; sprinkle with half the cheese. Repeat layers. Bake 15 minutes, or until the cheese is melted and the casserole is heated through. Break up the remaining tortillas and sprinkle over the casserole. Garnish with dollops of fat-free sour cream and sprinkle ½ cup chopped scallions over all.

TURKEY AND DRESSING

Cooking in an oven bag makes the turkey come out so moist and beautifully browned. It doesn't sit and swim in fat while cooking. The dressing is baked separately in a dressing pan or baking dish.

1 (8- to 12-pound) turkey
2 tablespoons flour

Dressing:
2 to 3 quarts crumbled dry fat-free corn bread
2 cups chopped onions
2 cups chopped celery
2 to 4 cups defatted turkey broth
2 to 4 tablespoons ground sage
Salt and pepper to taste
¾ cup egg substitute
Fat-free margarine or Butter Buds, liquid form

Giblet Gravy:
Reserved cooked giblets, chopped fine
1 cup uncooked dressing
3 tablespoons flour, or as needed
Defatted turkey broth

■ ■

Tip: (Buy turkey when prices are low or they are on sale; keep in freezer several weeks before holidays.) Three to four days ahead, take turkey out of freezer, place in an ice chest full of cold water, breast down, and change water approximately every 5 hours, keeping water cold. When thawed, drain and place in refrigerator. The size of your turkey will determine how far ahead you need to start this thawing process.

Turkey

Day ahead: Take turkey out of its original packing package, clean the neck and giblets, place in twice as much water as you need to cover the giblets, and boil until tender. When done, remove from the heat and cool. Cut giblets into small bite-size pieces for gravy. Place broth in the refrigerator overnight to defat. Store giblets in a zipper-lock plastic bag and refrigerate.

Trim all visible fat possible from the neck and tail area of turkey. Wash well in cold water. Drain.

Prepare a large (4 x 20-inch) oven bag by placing 2 tablespoons of flour in the bag and shaking to coat the inside. This will keep the turkey from sticking to the bag. Place a wire cake rack in the bottom of your roasting pan. (Don't forget to spray your roaster or roasting pan with vegetable oil cooking spray; it makes cleanup a snap.) (If you don't have a wire rack, you may use a pie plate or pan, turned upside down.) Place the turkey in the bag and tie as instructed on the package. Set the turkey, in its bag, on the rack or pan in the roaster. Place in refrigerator until time to cook. Before placing in the oven, punch holes in the bottom of the bag; this will let any excess fat drip out and into the pan. Also punch a few holes in the top of the bag, to let excess steam out. Cook according to directions on turkey timetable (included with turkey).

Dressing

Day ahead: Cook your corn bread. Clean and chop the onions and celery.

Day of preparation: Place onions and celery in a saucepan and cover with water. Cook until crisp-tender. Drain, reserving cooking water. Set aside.

Skim off any fat congealed on top of the broth and heat the broth to boiling. Preheat the oven to 350 degrees. Lightly spray your largest casserole with vegetable oil cooking spray.

In a big mixing bowl, combine the corn bread, sage, salt, and pepper. Add the celery and onions, using some of the water they were cooked in, and 2 cups of defatted broth. Stir until well blended. Don't add all your broth at once; add slowly, until desired consistency. Some like dressing drier than others.

Add the egg substitute and stir well. Pour into the prepared baking dish (reserve 1 cup for gravy) and dot with fat-free margarine or stream Butter Buds over the top. Bake, uncovered, about 30 to 45 minutes, until about half done; don't stir. Again add margarine or Butter Buds over top. Continue baking for another 30 to 45 minutes or until the desired doneness.

Giblet Gravy

Combine the giblets and defatted broth, about 4 cups, with 1 cup of uncooked dressing; bring to a boil and reduce heat. In a small bowl, mix about 3 tablespoons flour and 1 cup of hot broth with a small wire whisk or fork; when smooth, start adding to the gravy. Stir in a small amount at a time, until desired thickness. Remove from heat to stop thickening.

QUICK TURKEY POTPIE

2 (10¾-ounce) cans Healthy Request cream of mushroom soup
1 (16-ounce) package frozen mixed vegetables
3 cups cooked turkey or chicken, diced into small cubes
1 teaspoon poultry seasoning
½ teaspoon garlic salt
2 cups Bisquick reduced-fat baking mix
1½ cups skim milk
½ teaspoon parsley flakes

SERVES 8

3 GRAMS FAT
PER SERVING

Prep :25
Cook :35
Stand :00
Total 1:00

Preheat the oven to 400 degrees. Lightly spray a 13 x 9-inch baking pan with vegetable oil cooking spray.

In a large mixing bowl, combine the soup, vegetables, turkey, poultry seasoning, and garlic salt. Spoon into the prepared pan.

In a separate mixing bowl, stir together the baking mix and milk until blended. Pour over the turkey mixture. Sprinkle with parsley.

Bake uncovered 35 minutes or until the crust is light golden brown.

Leftover frozen or deli turkey or chicken can be used.

TURKEY, RICE, SAUSAGE, AND CRANBERRIES ALL IN ONE

Great for leftover holiday turkey, or make from scratch.

SERVES 8

LOW-FAT

Prep :20
Cook 1:20
Stand :00
Total 1:40

1 (6-ounce) package long grain and wild rice mix
½ pound lean bulk pork sausage (3 grams fat per patty)
1 cup sliced fresh mushrooms
½ cup chopped celery
1 tablespoon cornstarch
1 cup skim milk
3 cups chopped cooked turkey
1 cup dried cranberries or 1 (12-ounce) bag chopped fresh berries

Preheat the oven to 375 degrees. Lightly spray an 11 x 7-inch baking dish with vegetable oil cooking spray.

Prepare the rice according to package directions, omitting any butter, margarine, or salt. Set aside.

Dry-fry the sausage, mushrooms, and celery in a large nonstick skillet until the sausage is browned, stirring to crumble meat. Place in a colander and rinse with hot water; shake off excess water. Remove all but 1 teaspoon of pan drippings. In the skillet, place the cornstarch and gradually add the milk, stirring constantly with a wire whisk until the mixture is smooth and starts to thicken. Turn heat off.

Combine the rice, sausage mixture, sauce, turkey, and cranberries. Spoon the mixture into the prepared baking dish. Bake uncovered about 40 to 45 minutes.

To store: Cover and refrigerate up to 2 days. Or cover and freeze up to 2 weeks, thaw in refrigerator, and bake as directed above.

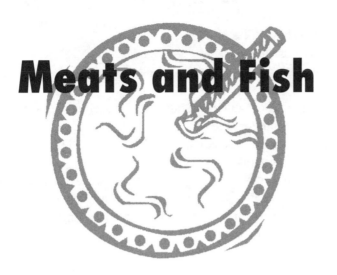

Meats and Fish

SNAKE MEAT

SERVES 4

**16 GRAMS FAT
ENTIRE DISH**

**Prep :15
Cook 2:00
Stand :00
Total 2:15**

1 (12-ounce) bottle chili sauce
1 (16-ounce) can cranberry sauce
1 (16-ounce) package low-fat Healthy Choice smoked sausage

In a large saucepan mix all ingredients together. Place over low heat and simmer for at least 2 hours.

I use a Crock-Pot and let it cook all day. Put it on before you leave in the morning. Great over rice.

Those girls in the hills really come up with some different dishes. Wait until you tell your friends what you are having for dinner when you invite them over. Makes me nervous when Jean invites us up into the hills for dinner.

POTATOES AND HAM AND PEAS IN A HURRY

SERVES 4

**4 GRAMS FAT
PER SERVING**

**Prep :05
Cook :14
Stand :00
Total :19**

This is my shortcut to a casserole-type dish made on top of the stove in a flash. Don't tell me you have no time to cook. Make your salad while this meal-in-one is cooking.

1 (24-ounce) package frozen hash-brown potatoes with peppers and onions
1½ cups cubed cooked 99% fat-free ham
1 (10¾-ounce) can Healthy Request cream of mushroom soup
1 cup frozen green peas
1 cup whole-kernel corn
½ teaspoon garlic salt
½ teaspoon Italian seasoning
Salt and pepper to taste

In a large nonstick skillet, combine the potatoes and ¾ cup of water. Bring to a boil, stirring often, reduce the heat, cover, and cook about 7 or 8 minutes or until the potatoes are tender. Stir in the ham, mushroom soup and half a soup can of water. Add the peas, corn, and seasonings. Cover and cook 5 to 6 minutes or until thoroughly heated, stirring occasionally.

CAJUN OVEN-FRIED FISH

This looks and tastes fried, but with no fat!
The types of fish may be catfish, grouper,
orange roughy, perch, bass, or just about any
type of fillets.

SERVES 6

ULTRA LOW-FAT

Prep :10
Cook :10
Stand :00
Total :20

½ cup cornmeal
½ cup dry bread crumbs
Dash of salt
1 teaspoon Cajun seasoning
1 pound fish fillets
⅔ cup skim milk or skim or low-fat buttermilk (1 gram per cup)

Preheat the oven to 450 degrees. Lightly spray a baking sheet with vegetable oil cooking spray.

Combine the cornmeal, bread crumbs, salt, and Cajun seasoning. Dip the fish in the skim milk or buttermilk and dredge in the cornmeal mixture. Place on the prepared baking sheet and spray the top of the fish lightly with cooking spray.

Bake for 10 minutes or until the fish flakes easily when tested with a fork. I usually turn mine over with a spatula after about half done. This makes it nice and brown on each side.

BOB'S "FRIED" FISH SPECIAL

SERVES 8

VERY LOW-FAT

Prep :10
Cook :20
Stand :00
Total :30

This may be done in a mixing bowl the same way, but this is the way Bob does it. He throws the bag away and there's no bowl to wash.

2 cups cornmeal
¼ cup Lemon pepper
1 teaspoon Creole seasoning
8 fish fillets

Preheat the oven to 400 degrees. Lightly spray a baking sheet with vegetable oil cooking spray.

In a small paper bag, mix the cornmeal, lemon pepper, and Creole seasoning. Rinse and drain the fish fillets. Put one or two fillets at a time in the paper bag and shake to coat evenly. Place on the baking sheet, spray the top of each piece lightly, and cook for about 20 minutes. Turn the fish when about half done.

Cheese, Rice, and Bean Dishes

GRILLED CHEESE SPECIAL

SERVES 2

1.5 GRAMS FAT PER SERVING

Prep :10
Cook :05
Stand :00
Total :15

1 tomato
1 onion
4 slices low-fat bread (less than 1 gram each)
Fat-free mayonnaise-type dressing
2 slices fat-free cheese

Slice the tomato and onion into thin slices. Spread each slice of bread on one side with mayonnaise. Put one slice of cheese on two of the slices, add slices of onion and tomato. Place the top of the sandwiches on; spray the bread lightly with vegetable oil cooking spray.

Spray a heated grill or nonstick skillet lightly with cooking spray. With a spatula place a sandwich in the skillet and brown slightly; turn sandwich over and brown on other side. Cut in half diagonally. Repeat with the remaining sandwich.

CHEESE ENCHILADAS

SERVES 8

1 GRAM FAT PER SERVING

Prep :20
Cook :25
Stand :00
Total :45

1 cup salsa
1½ cups fat-free cottage cheese
1 cup shredded fat-free Cheddar cheese
½ cup sliced scallions
¼ teaspoon crushed oregano
8 (6-inch) flour tortillas, warmed

Preheat the oven to 375 degrees. Spread ¼ cup salsa in the bottom of a 12 x 9-inch baking dish that has been lightly sprayed with vegetable oil cooking spray.

Combine the cottage cheese with ¼ cup Cheddar cheese, the scallions, and the oregano. Lay the tortillas on a work surface and spoon ¼ cup of the cottage cheese mixture down the center of each tortilla. Roll up and place seam side down over the salsa. Top with the remaining ¾ cup of Cheddar cheese and ¾ cup of salsa.

Cover with foil; bake for 20 to 25 minutes or until thoroughly heated.

Garnish with a few pieces of chopped green chiles.

CORNY CORNMEAL CASSEROLE

2 (16-ounce) cans cream-style corn
2 cups shredded fat-free Cheddar cheese
1 (4-ounce) can chopped green chiles
½ cup chopped onion
1 cup skim milk
½ cup egg substitute
1 cup yellow cornmeal
1½ teaspoons garlic salt
½ teaspoon baking soda

SERVES 8

0 GRAMS FAT

Prep :10
Cook :50
Stand :00
Total 1:00

Preheat the oven to 350 degrees. Lightly spray an 11 x 7-inch baking dish with vegetable oil cooking spray.

In a large mixing bowl, combine all ingredients, mixing until well blended. Pour into prepared baking dish.

Bake uncovered for about 50 minutes, or until a knife inserted in the center comes out clean.

VEGETARIAN FRIED RICE

SERVES 4

1 GRAM FAT PER 1-CUP SERVING

Prep :15
Cook :10
Stand: :00
Total :25

½ cup sliced scallions
¼ cup chopped green pepper
½ cup sliced fresh mushrooms
¼ cup shredded carrot
¼ teaspoon ground ginger
1 clove garlic, minced
3 cups cooked rice
2 tablespoons light soy sauce
¼ cup egg substitute
Dash pepper
¾ cup frozen green peas, thawed

Lightly spray a large nonstick skillet with vegetable oil cooking spray. Place over medium heat until just hot. Toss in the scallion slices, green pepper, mushrooms, carrot, ginger, and garlic. Cook and stir about 1 minute. Stir in rice and soy sauce. Lower the heat; cook while stirring occasionally with a fork for about 5 minutes.

Push the rice mixture to one side of the skillet. Add the egg substitute and pepper to the vacant spot; cook for about 4 minutes, stirring constantly. With a spatula, chop the egg mixture into small pieces. Add the peas to the rice and egg mixture, stirring gently to combine. Cook until thoroughly heated. Serve with additional soy sauce if desired.

RICE-STUFFED PEPPERS

Serve these hot, with a nice green salad on the same plate.

SERVES 4

0 GRAMS FAT

Prep :20
Cook :15
Stand :05
Total :40

2 cups fat-free chicken broth
1 cup raw rice
½ pound mushrooms, chopped
2 cloves garlic, minced
4 scallions, chopped (about 1 cup)
1 stalk celery with leaves, chopped
1 tablespoon fresh mixed herbs or 1 teaspoon dried (chives, oregano, dill,
   cilantro, tarragon, marjoram, or parsley)
8 ounces shredded fat-free Cheddar cheese
4 bell peppers, green, yellow, or red

In a large saucepan over high heat, bring the chicken broth to a boil. Add the rice and cook according to the directions on the package, leaving out the butter or margarine and salt. Drain and set aside.

In a microwave-safe dish lightly sprayed with vegetable oil cooking spray, mix the mushrooms and garlic. Cover and cook on high power for 8 minutes. Let stand covered for 2 minutes. Stir in scallions, celery, and herbs. Add the rice and shredded cheese. Toss to combine.

Slice the tops off the peppers very close to the top; remove membranes and seeds. Stuff the pepper cavities with the rice mixture. Place the peppers in a microwave-safe round or oval baking dish. Pour ½ cup water around the peppers, cover, and cook on high power for 8 minutes. Let stand covered 3 minutes. Serve hot.

RICE CASSEROLE

SERVES 8

1.25 GRAMS FAT PER SERVING

Prep :25
Cook :45
Stand :00
Total 1:10

2 (10¾-ounce) cans Healthy Request cream of broccoli soup
1 (8-ounce) can sliced water chestnuts, drained
1½ cups whole-kernel corn
Salt and pepper to taste
2 cups cooked rice

Preheat the oven to 350 degrees. Lightly spray an 8 x 10-inch baking dish with vegetable oil cooking spray.

In a large mixing bowl, combine the cream of broccoli soup, half a soup can of water, the water chestnuts, corn, salt, and pepper. Stir in the rice. Mix well.

Spoon into the prepared dish and bake uncovered for about 30 minutes.

EGGPLANT CASSEROLE

SERVES 6

0 GRAMS FAT

Prep :30
Cook 1:15
Stand :30
Total 2:15

1 medium eggplant, sliced into rounds ½ inch thick
1 teaspoon salt
1 cup uncooked rice
1 small onion, chopped
1 clove garlic, minced
2 cups sliced fresh mushrooms
1 (8-ounce) can tomato sauce
1 teaspoon dried oregano
½ teaspoon dried basil
2 cups fat-free cottage cheese
¼ cup skim milk
1 cup shredded fat-free mozzarella cheese

Spray a 2½-quart casserole or baking dish lightly with vegetable oil cooking spray.

Place the sliced eggplant in a bowl, add 1 teaspoon salt, then cover with water and soak about ½ hour. (This takes out the strong taste some eggplants have and helps prevent discoloring.)

Cook the rice in 2 cups water until tender; drain if necessary and set aside. Preheat the oven to 350 degrees.

Drain eggplant and steam until just tender. If you do not have a steamer, place ½ cup water in saucepan, add the eggplant, cover, and bring to a boil. Lower the heat and cook just until tender, with the lid on. Watch closely; the water might cook away and burn your eggplant.

In a nonstick skillet, sauté the onion, garlic, and mushrooms with ¼ cup water until they start to brown, stirring frequently. Add the tomato sauce, oregano, and basil.

In a small bowl, mix the cottage cheese and skim milk.

Assemble the casserole: Make a layer on the bottom with half the cooked rice. Top with half the eggplant, half the cottage cheese and milk mixture, half the mushroom tomato sauce, and half the mozzarella. Repeat, ending with the cheese.

Bake for 30 to 35 minutes or until bubbly and heated through.

QUICK BROCCOLI AND RICE

1 (16-ounce) package frozen broccoli
½ cup uncooked instant rice
½ cup skim milk
1 cup cubed cooked chicken breast
2 tablespoons fat-free Parmesan cheese

SERVES 2

1 GRAM FAT
PER SERVING

Prep :20
Cook 1:00
Stand :00
Total 1:20

Preheat the oven to 350 degrees. Lightly spray a 2-quart baking dish with vegetable oil cooking spray.

In a saucepan, cook the broccoli according to package directions. Drain.

Prepare the rice according to package directions, leaving out the butter or margarine and salt. *(continued)*

In a mixing bowl, combine the milk, broccoli, chicken, rice, and Parmesan cheese.

Pour into the prepared baking dish and bake uncovered for 25 to 30 minutes.

SAUSAGE BAKE

SERVES 6

VERY LOW-FAT

Prep :30
Cook 1:00
Stand :00
Total 1:30

1 pound low-fat sausage (3 grams per patty)
¾ cup chopped onion
½ cup chopped bell pepper
1 cup uncooked white rice
½ teaspoon lemon pepper
¼ teaspoon oregano
½ teaspoon adobo seasoning
¼ teaspoon dried basil
Salt and pepper to taste
1 (8-ounce) can sliced water chestnuts, drained
2 (10¾-ounce) cans Healthy Request cream of mushroom soup
1 (14-ounce) can fat-free chicken broth
1 (4-ounce) can mushroom pieces and stems, drained
1 (10-ounce) package frozen broccoli (run hot water over to thaw)

Preheat the oven to 350 degrees. Lightly coat a 13 x 9-inch baking dish with vegetable oil cooking spray.

Crumble and cook the sausage in a nonstick skillet. When the meat is about half done, add the onion and pepper. Cook 8 to 10 minutes, until tender. Blot any excess fat from the meat with paper towels.

Add the rice and all remaining ingredients. Pour into the prepared dish. Bake for 45 minutes to 1 hour, until the rice is tender and liquid is absorbed.

SAUSAGE BROCCOLI CASSEROLE

Serve this with a nice green salad and hot low-fat bread (no butter) and maybe corn for a side vegetable if desired.

SERVES 8

1.5 GRAMS FAT
PER 1-CUP
SERVING

Prep :20
Cook :55
Stand :00
Total 1:15

1 pound low-fat sage sausage (3 grams per patty), crumbled
½ cup chopped onion
½ cup chopped green pepper
1 (16-ounce) package chopped frozen broccoli, cooked until crisp-tender, drained
2 cups instant rice, prepared according to package directions, leaving out the butter or margarine and salt
2 (10¾-ounce) cans Healthy Request cream of broccoli soup
1 cup shredded fat-free Cheddar cheese
Pepper to taste

Preheat the oven to 350 degrees. Lightly spray a medium-size casserole with vegetable oil cooking spray.

Dry-fry the sausage in a large nonstick skillet, stirring to break up lumps, until browned and almost tender. Add the onion and green pepper when meat is about half cooked; sauté 5 minutes, stirring occasionally. Drain into a colander and rinse with hot water to remove any remaining fat. Blot with paper towels, return to the skillet, and add the broccoli, rice, soup, and ¾ soup can of water.

Bring to a simmer and stir in ¾ cup of the cheese. Transfer to the prepared casserole and sprinkle the remaining ¼ cup of cheese on top. Bake uncovered for 35 to 45 minutes, until lightly browned.

JAMBALAYA

This is a nice-size casserole for a crowd—or it can be cut in half.

SERVES 8

4.19 GRAMS FAT PER 1-CUP SERVING

Prep :35
Cook 1:10
Stand :00
Total 1:45

4 chicken breast halves, skin removed
1 (16-ounce) package Healthy Choice smoked sausage
1 (10¾-ounce) can French onion soup
1 (14-ounce) can vegetable broth
1 (10¾-ounce) can Healthy Request cream of celery soup
1 (14-ounce) can stewed tomatoes
1 (16-ounce) package Bayou Magic Cajun jambalaya rice mix (or any Cajun jambalaya rice mix)

Cover the chicken with water and boil 20 to 30 minutes, until tender. Debone and cut into 1-inch cubes. Defat the broth and reserve.

Preheat the oven to 350 degrees. Lightly spray a deep casserole or a 4-quart roasting pan with vegetable oil cooking spray.

Cut the sausage into 1-inch pieces and brown in a nonstick skillet. Pat off any excess fat with paper towels.

Mix together the onion soup, vegetable broth, celery soup, reserved chicken broth, and tomatoes. Before you add the rice from the package, put it in a strainer and, using *hot* water, rinse off some of the pepper seasoning; it is just too hot for us Okies. (If you live in Cajun country, add just as is.) I reserve the water in a bowl with the seasoning to make sure it has enough; if not hot enough, add some of the Cajun-seasoned water. Don't run too much water over the rice—just about 2 cups.

Add the chopped meats to the above mixture, place in the prepared casserole, and bake for 30 to 35 minutes, until all the rice is tender.

SMOKED SAUSAGE, BEANS, AND RICE

Most sausage, bean, and rice dishes take half a day to cook; this one takes half an hour.

SERVES 6

2 GRAMS FAT
PER SERVING

Prep :15
Cook :32
Stand :00
Total :47

1 pound low-fat smoked sausage such as Healthy Choice (1.5 grams fat per 2 ounces), sliced and each slice quartered

¾ cup chopped onion (may use frozen)

½ cup chopped green pepper (may use frozen)

¾ cup chopped celery

1 tablespoon chopped garlic, prepared or fresh

1 (16-ounce) can fat-free refried beans with salsa, such as Rosarita

2 (15-ounce) cans ranch-style pinto beans, undrained

½ cup medium or hot prepared salsa

4 drops hot sauce, or to taste

1 tablespoon Cajun spice

1 teaspoon chili powder

2 cups instant rice, prepared according to package directions, leaving out the butter or margarine and salt

In a large deep nonstick skillet, brown the sausage; add the onions, green peppers, celery, and garlic. Add about ¼ cup water and sauté over medium heat for 5 to 7 minutes or until the vegetables are tender. If using frozen vegetables you may not need to add as much water.

Pour in 1 cup of water, the refried beans, and the 2 cans of pinto beans; stir until well mixed. (Refried beans will thicken your dish; water is to make a nice consistency. You may need to add a little more, according to your own preference.)

Add the salsa, hot sauce, Cajun spice, and chili powder. Stir to mix. Simmer the dish for about 10 minutes, add the rice, and mix well. Continue to simmer for 5 to 10 minutes, until hot.

OKLAHOMA LAZY DAZE
TEX-MEX CASSEROLE

SERVES 6

1.5 GRAMS FAT
ENTIRE DISH

Prep :20
Cook :50
Stand :00
Total 1:10

1 (14-ounce) can stewed tomatoes, undrained
1 (16-ounce) can fat-free refried beans
1 (16-ounce) can fat-free vegetable chili
1 (4-ounce) can chopped green chiles
2 cups yellow cornmeal
1 (16-ounce) can chili beans
½ cup chopped onion
1 cup shredded fat-free Cheddar cheese
1 cup crushed baked low-fat tortilla chips (1 gram fat per 13 chips)
1 cup commercial salsa
¾ cup chopped scallions, tops and all, plus more as needed
1 cup fat-free sour cream (optional)
Optional garnish: chopped lettuce, chopped tomatoes, carrot sticks, celery sticks

Preheat the oven to 350 degrees. Lightly spray a deep casserole or baking dish with vegetable oil cooking spray.

Pour the tomatoes, juice and all, into the baking dish. Spoon refried beans on top of the tomatoes, spreading to make a fairly even layer. Pour the vegetable chili over the refried bean layer. Spread the green chiles over all.

In a separate bowl, mix the cornmeal and 1½ cups boiling water, making a mushy consistency. (You may need to add a little more water.) Spread this mixture over the green chiles. Pour the chili beans over the cornmeal mixture. Spread chopped onion over the chili beans; sprinkle shredded cheese over onions.

Bake uncovered for 40 to 50 minutes. Sprinkle crushed chips over all. Pour salsa over the chips, sprinkle on the chopped scallions, and dollop sour cream over all, if desired.

To serve, make a nice circle of chopped lettuce around the outside of each dinner plate; place a serving of the casserole in the center of the plate, and garnish the lettuce ring with tomatoes. Place a couple of carrot sticks and celery sticks alongside the lettuce. Makes a very pretty plate and meal in one.

COOKING FOR MY KIDS

Let me tell you about cooking for my five kids.

I have one boy and one girl. Bob has three boys. I already had my two children when we got married. We were only married six weeks when the first of his boys came to live with us, and within six months we had them all. *All five.* Wow! I was only thirty-two. Can you just imagine a thirty-two-year-old with five kids, ages eleven, twelve, thirteen, fourteen, and fifteen? Neither can I.

We had a normal three-bedroom house with seven people living in it. I had the furniture taken out of the dining room to put beds in. We then cleaned out the garage, paneled, carpeted, and fixed it all up with black lights, and all the beads and junk that were so popular at that time. We bought four twin-size beds and now had our own dormitory. I was all set up to run this institution.

We had a very good group of kids. We really got a lot of attention when we went places with these five, looking like the Brady Bunch. Remember that TV show? Well, this was the Rohde Bunch.

The boys played football, wrestled, and did all the things that seemed to create appetites that teenage boys do not need any help creating.

My friends would ask me, "How do you cook for that bunch?" My reply: "In a big pot." I would think nothing of cooking four pounds of bacon and two dozen eggs and making thirty-six big homemade biscuits for a Saturday breakfast, plus a big bowl of gravy.

I would come home from work and fry two large chickens, cook eight to ten pounds of potatoes, four cans of green beans, four cans of corn, and a large pan of corn bread and never even bat an eye. During that time I would be shouting orders left and right, doing forty tons of laundry, and picking up the place as I awaited the arrival of my Bob. Now I am out of breath at the thought. Youth!

As luck would have it, these four new men I had to feed would eat anything if it didn't crawl off the plate before they could stab it. They liked my cooking so much, that it got to the point where I had to limit each one. I would fill the platters with what I had figured as portion sizes and set them on the table, all the while shouting out limitations. Each kid could have three pieces of this, two of that, one of this, and so forth down the line. If anyone would reach for his not-commissioned piece of food, I would jokingly pretend to stab their hand with my fork. We couldn't buy enough milk to satisfy their undying thirst—we had to limit them to one gallon a day. We had a milk delivery man at that time. He loved us.

We had a lot of fun and a lot of discipline. We got through it, penniless, alive, and well. Five graduated from school. Bob and I graduated into an empty nest.

Those were the young days of grease and cholesterol. Well, now we pay the price. No more of that. I wish that I had been as fat-smart as I am now so that I could have cooked a much healthier meal for those human garbage disposals. Their pipes would have been much better off. By the way, Bob is a mechanical engineer (plumbing, heating, air conditioning). I'll tell you how I met him in another story. Feeding this group is a story all of its own. You should have seen us go to the grocery story once a week. Oh, my!

QUICK-THE-KIDS-ARE-COMING CASEROLE

(Throw Something in the Pot)

SERVES 8

2 GRAMS FAT PER SERVING

Prep :25
Cook 1:30
Stand :00
Total 1:55

8 ounces low-fat smoked sausage (such as Healthy Choice), sliced and each slice quartered
2 medium-size onions, halved lengthwise, sliced thin
6 boneless skinless chicken tenders, cut into 1½-inch pieces
1 tablespoon minced garlic
Pinch of oregano
Pinch of dried basil
½ teaspoon pepper
1 (16-ounce) can tomatoes, undrained
¾ cup dry white wine or canned fat-free chicken broth
3 (16-ounce) cans white beans, rinsed and drained (sometimes I mix two or three kinds of beans, whatever I have on hand)
2 cups coarse fresh bread crumbs (can use dried crumbs)

Preheat the oven to 325 degrees. Lightly spray a 4-quart casserole with vegetable oil cooking spray.

Dry-fry the sausage and onions in a nonstick skillet, stirring occasionally, for 5 to 7 minutes, until onions are translucent. Add the chicken, garlic, oregano, basil, and pepper. Cook 5 minutes or so, until the chicken is tender. Add the tomatoes and the wine. Bring to a boil and boil about 3 minutes. Stir in the beans. Spoon the mixture into the prepared casserole. Cover with foil and bake for 1 hour.

Prepare the crumb mixture: Place crumbs in a mixing bowl and spray lightly with cooking spray; stir and spray again; stir and spray again until very lightly coated.

Uncover the casserole, sprinkle the crumb mixture over evenly, and continue to bake for 30 additional minutes or until the crumbs are lightly browned.

Note: If making ahead, cook 1 hour, remove cover, and cool 30 to 40 minutes. Refrigerate uncovered until cool. Cover and refrigerate up to 3 days. When ready to serve, remove cover, top with crumb mixture, and bake 30 to 40 minutes or until the crumbs are browned and the casserole is heated through.

MEXICAN BEAN PIE

SERVES 6

2.3 GRAMS FAT
PER SERV-
ING—⅙ OF
PIE

Prep :15
Cook :30
Stand :15
Total 1:00

Crust:
1½ cups yellow cornmeal
¼ teaspoon salt (optional)
2 teaspoons canola oil
½ to ¾ cup hot water, or more as needed

Filling:
1 (16-ounce) can fat-free refried beans
½ cup commercial salsa, green or red
1½ cups cooked rice
2 scallions, chopped fine
1 tablespoon chopped cilantro leaves
1 (4-ounce) can chopped green chiles
¼ cup shredded fat-free Monterey Jack cheese

Preheat the oven to 350 degrees.

Combine the cornmeal and salt, if desired, in a mixing bowl. Add the oil, blend with a fork, and stir in enough hot water so that a dough forms, pulling away from sides of bowl and balling up in the center.

Spray a 9-inch pie plate lightly with vegetable oil cooking spray. Press the dough evenly on the bottom and sides, pinching a finished edge around top. If time allows, chill before filling. (The pie crust may be made ahead of time and filled at the last minute.)

Spread ⅓ of the beans over the bottom of the crust. Spread 1 to 2 tablespoons of salsa over the bean layer.

Toss the rice with the scallions and cilantro. Spread evenly over bean layer and pat gently to pack just a tiny bit. Make a layer of the chiles on top of the rice. Layer the remaining beans and salsa over the chiles.

Bake uncovered 25 to 30 minutes, sprinkling the cheese over the pie for the last 5 minutes of baking time. Let stand 15 minutes before slicing.

Garnish with fat-free sour cream and a slice of avocado and a slice of tomato for your salad on the side. Here you have your bread, vegetables, dairy, and salad all in one dish.

QUICK CHILI

3 cups chopped onion
1 carrot, chopped
1 teaspoon minced jalapeño
3 to 4 teaspoons chili powder
1 teaspoon minced garlic, prepared or fresh
1½ teaspoons ground cumin
3 (14-ounce) cans stewed tomatoes, undrained
2 (16-ounce) cans kidney or chili beans, drained
⅓ cup fine- or medium-grain bulgur

SERVES 4

0 GRAMS FAT

Prep :20
Cook :28
Stand :00
Total :48

In a heavy nonstick dutch oven or saucepan, heat ¼ cup of water; add the onions, carrot, jalapeño, chili powder, garlic, and cumin. Sauté for 5 to 8 minutes, or until the onions and carrots are soft.

Add the tomatoes with their juice, the beans, and the bulgur. Cook for 5 more minutes and reduce the heat to low. Simmer the chili uncovered for 15 minutes or until thickened.

VEGETABLE CHILI

SERVES 6

0 GRAMS FAT

Prep :25
Cook :50
Stand :00
Total 1:15

If you like your chili just a little hotter you might like to experiment with this and add 1½ or 2 packages of chili seasoning. My brother says chili isn't hot unless it makes the top of your bald head itch.

1 cup coarsely chopped onion
1 medium green bell pepper, chopped coarse
1 cup chopped celery
2 cloves garlic, minced
1 (14-ounce) can stewed tomatoes, undrained
1 (15-ounce) can white beans or Great Northern beans
2 (16-ounce) cans chili-seasoned beans
2 (11-ounce) cans white shoepeg corn
1 (4-ounce) can chopped green chiles
1 (15-ounce) can tomato sauce
1 (1.25-ounce) package chili seasoning mix (such as McCormick)

In a deep nonstick saucepan or skillet, sauté the onion, pepper, celery, and garlic in ¼ cup water for 5 minutes or until softened. Stir frequently to keep garlic from burning.

Add the tomatoes, juice and all, the beans, corn, green chiles, and tomato sauce. Stir to mix ingredients well. Stir in the chili seasoning, mixing well. Lower the heat and simmer for 30 to 45 minutes.

CHILI VEGETABLE STEW

2½ cups chopped zucchini
3⅓ cups chopped green pepper
¾ cup chopped onions
1 (1¾-ounce) package chili seasoning mix
1 (15-ounce) can kidney beans, undrained
1 (15-ounce) can tomato sauce
1 (7-ounce) can whole-kernel corn, drained
2 cups uncooked instant rice

SERVES 6

LESS THAN 0.5
GRAM FAT PER
SERVING

Prep :20
Cook :20
Stand :05
Total :45

In a large nonstick skillet, sauté the zucchini, peppers, and onions in ¼ cup of water for 5 to 8 minutes, until crisp-tender. Add the seasoning mix and stir in 2 cups of water, the beans, and tomato sauce. Bring to a boil. Lower the heat to a simmer and cook for 10 more minutes, stirring occasionally.

Stir in the corn. (I like shoepeg corn the best, but regular corn is fine), return to a boil, stir in rice, and cover. Remove from heat. Let stand for about 5 minutes. Serve with shredded cheese, chopped onions, sour cream, and salsa.

HAM AND BEANS (WITHOUT THE FAT)

Ham hock, or chunk of ham
2 pounds white navy or brown pinto beans

SERVES 8

0 GRAMS FAT

Prep :15
Cook 3:30
Stand :00
Total 3:45

The day before bean cooking day, place the ham hock in a large stockpot, cover with water, and simmer until tender, about 1½ hours. Remove the ham from the stock, let cool. Refrigerate the stock overnight; all the fat will collect to the top and congeal; you can just lift it off and throw it away. (I have often thought of getting into the refrigerator overnight myself and seeing if I would congeal enough to lift off a couple or three pounds from several unsightly areas.) *(continued)*

Look over the beans carefully for bits of dirt and pebbles, and wash thoroughly. Place in a deep stockpot or dutch oven, cover with the defatted stock, and bring to a boil. Lower the heat to a slow boil, cooking ½ to 2 hours or until the beans are tender and the liquid has thickened.

You may add lean chunks of ham if desired, but this will add fat grams, and you already have the flavor from the broth. If you are adding the ham, do so when beans are about half done.

Some people like to wash their beans and soak them overnight before cooking. I have heard arguments both ways. You write and tell me. I personally do not soak my beans ahead of time.

SHORTCUT BEANS AND RICE

SERVES 4

LESS THAN 1 GRAM FAT PER SERVING

Prep :20
Cook :10
Stand :00
Total :30

½ cup thinly sliced scallions
1 (8-ounce) can tomato sauce
1 (14-ounce) can spicy chili beans, undrained
½ teaspoon dried basil
2 cloves garlic, minced
½ teaspoon Cajun seasoning (more may be added according to your desired temperature)
2½ cups cooked rice

In a nonstick skillet, sauté the scallions in about ¼ cup water for about 2 minutes. Add the tomato sauce, beans, basil, and garlic. Stir in the Cajun seasoning, using the "add and taste" method until desired spiciness is reached. Simmer about 4 minutes and add the cooked rice, stirring until thoroughly heated.

> *Variation:* This may be made ahead according to the above instructions, placed in a baking dish, covered with plastic wrap, and refrigerated. Remove plastic wrap and heat in the oven at 350 degrees for 20 to 25 minutes, until thoroughly heated, or microwave on high for 4 to 6 minutes, stirring twice during the heating period.

BEAN BURRITOS

8 (6-inch) flour tortillas
1 cup chopped onion
1 (16-ounce) can fat-free refried beans
1 (4-ounce) can diced green chiles, drained
4 dashes hot pepper sauce
¾ cup salsa
1½ cups shredded fat-free cheddar cheese
For garnish: fat-free sour cream, diced fresh tomato, diced green chiles

SERVES 8

1 GRAM FAT
PER SERVING

Prep :20
Cook :25
Stand :00
Total :45

Stack tortillas one on top of the other, wrap in foil, and heat in the oven at 350 degrees for about 10 minutes.

In a nonstick skillet, sauté the onion in 2 tablespoons of water for 5 minutes or until tender. Do not drain. Add the refried beans, green chiles, and hot pepper sauce. Cook and stir until heated through.

Spoon about ⅓ cup of the bean mixture onto each tortilla just down the center. Spoon about 1½ tablespoons of salsa over the bean mixture. Sprinkle about 3 tablespoons of cheese over the salsa. Roll up the tortilla and place on a foil-lined cooking sheet. Bake loosely covered in a 350-degree oven for about 10 minutes, or until thoroughly heated.

Serve with a dollop of fat-free sour cream, some diced fresh tomato, and diced green chiles if desired.

SPICY BEAN BURRITO EXPRESS

SERVES 2

1 GRAM FAT PER SERVING

Prep :20
Cook :28
Stand :00
Total :48

1 (16-ounce) can fat-free refried beans
4 (8-inch) flour tortillas
1½ cups shredded fat-free Cheddar cheese
4 tablespoons chopped onion
1 (10-ounce) can red enchilada sauce
¼ cup fat-free sour cream
½ cup salsa

Preheat the oven to 350 degrees. Lightly spray an 8-inch square pan with vegetable oil cooking spray.

Spoon ¼ of the refried beans into the center of each tortilla. Sprinkle each with ¼ cup cheese and a tablespoon of the onion. Roll each tortilla, fold the ends under, and place seam side down in the prepared pan. Pour enchilada sauce over the burritos; cover the pan with foil.

Bake at 350 degrees for 25 minutes. Uncover, sprinkle with remaining cheese, and return to the oven for an additional 2 or 3 minutes, until the cheese is melted. Serve with sour cream and salsa.

BEAN BURRITO CASSEROLE

SERVES 4

LOW-FAT

Prep :25
Cook 1:10
Stand :00
Total 1:35

*Great make-ahead dish. Oh! This is so good
and so good for you.*

8 (8-inch) flour tortillas
½ pound lean ground turkey
1½ cups tomato juice
1 (1¼-ounce) package taco seasoning mix
1 (16-ounce) can fat-free refried beans
2 cups shredded fat-free Cheddar cheese
For garnish: shredded lettuce, chopped tomato, sliced scallions, fat-free sour
    cream, commercial salsa

Preheat the oven to 350 degrees. Lightly spray a 13 x 9-inch baking dish with vegetable oil cooking spray.

Stack the tortillas, wrap in foil, and place in the oven for 10 minutes, or until warmed and workable. (You can also dip them in hot water one at a time and pat dry if you're in a hurry, as I always am.)

Brown the turkey in a nonstick skillet, stirring to crumble. Meanwhile, in a saucepan, combine the tomato juice and seasoning mix, bring to a boil, reduce heat, and simmer about 5 minutes while turkey is cooking. Transfer the cooked turkey to a colander, rinse with hot water, and shake excess water off. Return to skillet (wipe the skillet with paper towels to rid of any fat). Stir in the beans and half the tomato juice mixture.

To assemble: Place ¼ cup of the turkey mixture down the center of each tortilla. Roll up the tortillas and place seam side down in the prepared baking dish and top with 2 tablespoons of cheese.

To store: If making ahead, cover with plastic wrap at this point, and refrigerate up to 8 hours. Refrigerate the remaining tomato juice mixture in a tightly covered container.

To bake and serve: Pour the remaining juice over the casserole, cover with foil, and bake at 350 degrees for 35 to 40 minutes. Uncover, sprinkle with the remaining cheese, and bake an additional 5 minutes or until the cheese melts.

Serving suggestions: Make a circle of shredded lettuce around your plate about 2 inches wide. Layer with a ring of chopped tomatoes; top with scallions. Sprinkle cheese over for more color if desired. Place 2 burritos in the center of each. Dollop fat-free sour cream on burritos if desired.

Pasta and Pizza

PASTA TIPS

Pasta is easy to cook, but you should pay attention because it is also easy to have a "pot of paste" if you aren't following the basics. Use a large pot and plenty of water. The pasta needs room to move and circulate.

Bring the water to a rapid boil before you add the pasta. A lid on the pot will hold the heat and help the water to boil faster.

Add the pasta slowly. If it is short pasta, such as macaroni, stir the boiling water with a long-handled spoon as you add the pasta. When cooking long pasta, such as spaghetti, hold a handful at one end and gradually bend the pasta around the inside of the pot as it softens. Stir now and then so the pasta doesn't stick together or settle in a lump on the bottom. A lump of pasta is nothing to write home about, for sure. Keep the pasta moving and the pot *un*covered. Adjust the heat so the pasta keeps boiling and moving, but not so high that it boils over.

Follow the recommended cooking time on the package, but check two or three minutes before to make sure you don't overcook. Remove a piece of pasta, rinse with cold water to keep from burning your mouth, and bite into it. Perfect pasta should be slightly firm in the center. If it's not quite done, check again in a minute or two. If the pasta is to be used in a casserole and cooked again, cook it slightly firmer than pasta to be eaten right away.

Pour the pasta into a colander set in the sink. Shake the colander gently to drain off excess water. If the pasta is to be eaten right away, just drain and serve. If it is to be used in a salad or such, rinse with cold water to stop the cooking. Pasta can be cooked ahead of time, drained, and stored in a plastic bag or bowl in the refrigerator until it's needed.

FETTUCCINE

8 ounces uncooked wide no-egg noodles
1 cup fat-free cottage cheese, at room temperature (see Note)
½ cup fat-free Parmesan cheese
Salt and pepper to taste (optional)
¼ cup minced fresh parsley

Boil the noodles according to package directions. Drain and return to the same pot. Quickly toss together with the remaining ingredients. Serve immediately.

Note: I mash my cottage cheese a little to avoid larger lumps.

SERVES 4

0.5 GRAM FAT
PER SERVING

Prep :10
Cook :10
Stand :00
Total :20

SPICY ANGEL HAIR PASTA

1 medium onion, sliced thin
1 clove garlic, minced
1 (28-ounce) can tomatoes, coarsely chopped or crushed
2 tablespoons minced fresh cilantro
Few drops of hot pepper sauce, or to taste
¼ teaspoon salt (optional)
¼ teaspoon sugar (optional)
12 ounces uncooked angel hair pasta
Grated fat-free Parmesan cheese (optional)

In a large heavy saucepan, over medium heat, sauté the onion and garlic in about ¼ cup of water. Sauté until tender, stirring constantly. Be careful not to burn the garlic.

Add the tomatoes, cilantro, hot pepper sauce, salt, and sugar, if desired. Bring to a slow boil, reduce the heat to low, and simmer uncovered for about 30 minutes, or until slightly thickened.

While the sauce is cooking, prepare the pasta according to pack-

SERVES 4

LESS THAN 1
GRAM FAT PER
SERVING

Prep :15
Cook :45
Stand :00
Total 1:00

age directions, leaving out any oil or margarine called for. Drain. Transfer to a heated platter and keep warm.

To serve, spoon the sauce over the pasta and sprinkle with Parmesan cheese.

PASTA ROLL-UPS

A good make-ahead dish. Make it one day and cook the next, or freeze and bake when desired.

SERVES 4

1 GRAM FAT
PER ROLL-UP

Prep :25
Cook 1:20
Stand :00
Total 1:45

1 large onion, chopped fine
1 teaspoon crumbled dried basil
½ teaspoon crumbled dried marjoram
2 cloves garlic, minced
½ teaspoon black pepper
1 boneless skinless chicken breast half, chopped fine (about 8 ounces)
1 (26-ounce) jar fat-free pizza sauce
8 uncooked lasagne noodles, ruffle-edge type (for prettier appearance)
½ (10-ounce) package frozen chopped spinach, thawed and drained (squeeze out all water possible)
½ cup grated fat-free Parmesan cheese
1 cup fat-free cottage cheese

In a nonstick skillet, sauté the onion, basil, marjoram, half the garlic, and half the pepper until the onion is soft, about 3 to 5 minutes. Remove 2 tablespoons and set aside.

Add the chopped chicken to the skillet and cook, stirring, for 4 minutes. Reduce the heat to low and add the pizza sauce. Cook uncovered for 15 to 20 minutes, stirring occasionally. Set aside.

Meanwhile, cook the lasagne noodles according to package directions, omitting salt and oil if called for. Rinse and drain.

Preheat the oven to 375 degrees. Lightly spray a 9 x 9-inch baking dish with vegetable oil cooking spray.

For the filling, in a medium-size bowl combine the spinach with ¼ cup of the Parmesan cheese and all the cottage cheese. Add the remaining garlic and pepper, and the reserved onion mixture. Mix well.

Spoon half the tomato sauce into the prepared baking dish. Spread 3 tablespoons or so of the cheese filling on each noodle, roll up as you would a jelly roll, and place seam side down in the baking dish. Repeat until all the noodles are used. Top with the remaining sauce.

Cover with foil and bake for 25 to 30 minutes. Uncover, sprinkle the remaining Parmesan cheese on top, and bake uncovered 5 to 6 minutes longer.

TEX-MEX LASAGNE

1 (14-ounce) can fat-free chili, with or without beans
1 (16-ounce) jar Mexican salsa, drained
1 (4-ounce) can mushroom stems and pieces, drained
¾ cup grated fat-free Parmesan cheese
1½ teaspoons Italian seasoning
1½ cups fat-free cottage cheese
1½ teaspoons parsley flakes
9 cooked lasagne noodles
2½ cups shredded fat-free mozzarella cheese

SERVES 6

1 GRAM FAT
PER SERVING

Prep : 20
Cook: 40
Stand : 10
Total 1:10

Preheat the oven to 350 degrees. Lightly spray a 9 x 9-inch baking dish with vegetable oil cooking spray.

Combine the chili, drained salsa, mushroom pieces, Parmesan cheese, and Italian seasoning. In a small bowl, combine the cottage cheese and parsley flakes.

Line the bottom of the prepared baking dish with ⅓ of the noodles. Dot with ⅓ of the cottage cheese. Spread evenly with ⅓ of the chili mixture and sprinkle with ⅓ of the mozzarella. Repeat to make three layers.

Bake uncovered for 30 to 40 minutes, or until the lasagne is thoroughly heated. Let stand 10 minutes before serving.

SPAGHETTI PIZZA

SERVES 8

2 GRAMS FAT PER SERVING

Prep :25
Cook :40
Stand :05
Total 1:10

½ cup skim milk
¼ cup egg substitute
4 cups cooked spaghetti
½ pound ground lean turkey
1 cup chopped onion
1 cup chopped green bell pepper
2 cloves garlic, minced
1 (15-ounce) can tomato sauce
1 teaspoon Italian seasoning
1 teaspoon salt-free herb seasoning
¼ teaspoon pepper
1 cup sliced mushrooms
2 cups shredded fat-free Cheddar and mozzarella cheese mixed

Preheat the oven to 350 degrees. Lightly spray a 15 x 10-inch jelly roll pan with vegetable oil cooking spray.

In a medium-size mixing bowl, blend the milk and egg substitute. Add the cooked spaghetti and toss to coat. Spread the spaghetti mixture evenly in the prepared pan. Set aside.

In a large nonstick skillet, cook the turkey, onion, green pepper, and garlic until the turkey is done. Add the tomato sauce and seasonings; simmer 5 minutes. Spoon the meat mixture evenly over the spaghetti. Top with mushrooms and cheese. Bake uncovered 20 to 25 minutes. Let stand 5 minutes before cutting.

Variation: Use lean ground pork or beef in place of the ground turkey.

PIZZA CRUST

1 tablespoon sugar
1 envelope (¼ ounce) fast-rising dry yeast
1 cup warm water
3 cups all-purpose flour
2 teaspoons olive oil
¼ teaspoon salt
1 tablespoon cornmeal

SERVES 2

14 GRAMS FAT
ENTIRE CRUST

Prep :15
Cook :00
Stand :55
Total 1:10

In a large mixing bowl, dissolve sugar and yeast in warm water; let stand 5 minutes. Add 2¾ cups of the flour, the oil, and salt, mixing until a soft dough forms.

Turn the dough out onto a lightly floured surface. Knead until smooth, about 10 minutes. Add enough of the remaining flour, 1 tablespoon at a time, to prevent dough from sticking to hands.

Place the dough in a bowl coated with vegetable oil cooking spray. Spray the top lightly. Cover with a damp kitchen towel and let rise in a warm place about 30 minutes or until doubled in bulk.

Lightly coat two 12-inch pizza pans or baking sheets with cooking spray and sprinkle each with 1½ teaspoons cornmeal.

Punch down dough and divide in half. Roll each half into a 12-inch circle on a lightly floured surface. (I sometimes use a cookie sheet if I am having guests and need a larger pizza.) Place the dough in the prepared pans. Cover and let rise 20 additional minutes.

Uncover the dough and prepare pizza according to directions. (Use the standing time to get your fresh veggies pared and ready for your topping.)

COUNTRY PIZZA

SERVES 4

0 GRAMS FAT

Prep :20
Cook :50
Stand :00
Total 1:10

1½ cups yellow cornmeal
½ teaspoon salt (optional)
1 to 1½ cups boiling water
2 tablespoons grated fat-free Parmesan cheese
1 (26-ounce) jar fat-free pizza sauce
2 cups shredded fat-free mozzarella cheese
Chopped onion, chopped green pepper, drained canned sliced mushrooms, drained canned beans, or other desired toppings
Crumbled dried basil (optional)
Dried oregano (optional)

Preheat the oven to 350 degrees.

In a medium mixing bowl, combine the cornmeal and salt, if desired. Gradually add the boiling water, stirring with a fork, until it is thick and forms a soft ball (not mushy). Add the Parmesan cheese; mix well.

With wet hands, pat the cornmeal mixture evenly into a 23-inch pizza pan or baking sheet lightly sprayed with vegetable oil cooking spray.

Bake the crust uncovered for 15 minutes or until just golden.

Spread the sauce evenly over the crust and sprinkle with half the mozzarella. Add your choice of vegetables and toppings, and additional sauce if desired; sprinkle with herbs and top with the remaining cheese.

Bake uncovered 10 to 15 minutes or until the cheese has melted. Cut into wedges.

> *Note:* If you like your vegetables a little softer, sauté them in a nonstick skillet for a few minutes; you may want to add about ⅛ cup water, but usually the onion and pepper have enough water in them to do the job.

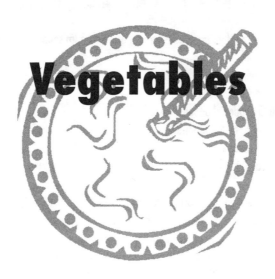

Vegetables

GREEN BEAN CASSEROLE

SERVES 6

4 GRAMS FAT
ENTIRE DISH

Prep :15
Cook :45
Stand :00
Total 1:00

1 (10¾-ounce) can Healthy Request cream of mushroom soup
1¼ cups skim milk
2 (14-ounce) cans green beans, drained
2 medium onions, chopped
1 medium bell pepper, chopped
Salt and pepper to taste (optional)
¼ cup fine dry bread crumbs
1 teaspoon grated fat-free Parmesan cheese

Preheat the oven to 350 degrees.

Mix soup and milk. Mix drained green beans with chopped onion and bell pepper. Place in a baking dish lightly sprayed with vegetable oil cooking spray. Pour the soup mixture over. Add salt and pepper if desired. Top with bread crumbs and Parmesan cheese. Bake for 40 to 45 minutes or until nice and bubbly and lightly browned.

GREEN BEANS ITALIANO

SERVES 4

0 GRAMS FAT

Prep :10
Cook :10
Stand :00
Total :20

1 quart green beans, or 1 (10-ounce) package frozen may be used (I can my own)
1 (14-ounce) can Italian tomatoes, drained and chopped
¼ cup chopped onion
1 clove garlic, chopped fine
½ teaspoon dried oregano leaves (1 teaspoon fresh)
½ teaspoon dried basil leaves (1 teaspoon fresh)
⅛ teaspoon pepper

Combine all the ingredients in a saucepan and heat to boiling; reduce heat. Cover and simmer 8 to 10 minutes, or until the beans are crisp-tender. (Some of you like your green beans softer, so cook according to your desired taste.)

BROCCOLI CASSEROLE

½ cup chopped onion
½ cup chopped celery
1 (16-ounce) package frozen broccoli, thawed
1 (10¾-ounce) can Healthy Request cream of chicken soup
¾ cup skim milk
1 cup uncooked instant rice, or more if desired
3 cups shredded fat-free Cheddar cheese

SERVES 6

4 GRAMS FAT
ENTIRE DISH

Prep :15
Cook :45
Stand :00
Total 1:00

Preheat the oven to 350 degrees. Spray a casserole or a 13 x 9-inch baking dish lightly with vegetable oil cooking spray.

Sauté the onion and celery in ¼ cup of water in a medium saucepan until hot and bubbly. Add 1 cup of water; bring to a boil and add broccoli. Cover and let cook for about 10 minutes over low heat.

Stir in the soup, milk, and rice (adding more liquid if you use additional rice). Bring to a boil. Transfer to the prepared casserole and top with the cheese. Bake uncovered for 20 to 30 minutes, until the cheese is golden brown.

CORN AND BROCCOLI

1 (10-ounce) package frozen broccoli cuts, thawed, or 1½ cups fresh broccoli florets
1 cup frozen whole-kernel corn, thawed
½ cup water
½ cup chopped onion
2 teaspoons chopped fresh basil or ½ teaspoon dried basil
½ teaspoon vegetable bouillon granules
1 clove garlic, chopped fine
1 (2-ounce) jar diced pimentos, drained

SERVES 4

0 GRAMS FAT

Prep :10
Cook :12
Stand :00
Total :22

Heat all ingredients to boiling, reduce the heat, cover, and simmer for 4 to 5 minutes (10 to 12 minutes if using fresh broccoli), or until broccoli is crisp-tender.

SQUASH CASSEROLE

Cook one and freeze one for later. The squash are plentiful in the summertime, so you'll have a quick meal ready later when they are all gone.

SERVES 10

VERY LOW-FAT

Prep :20
Cook :52
Stand :00
Total 1:12

1 package herb-seasoned stuffing mix
1 cup Butter Buds, liquid form (see Note)
1 to 1½ pounds yellow squash, sliced
2 small onions, chopped
1 (10¾-ounce) can Healthy Request cream of chicken soup
1 pint fat-free sour cream.
1 (4-ounce) jar pimentos, drained and chopped
1 (4-ounce) can sliced water chestnuts, drained
2 cups grated fat-free Cheddar cheese

Preheat the oven to 350 degrees. Lightly spray two 1½-quart casserole dishes with vegetable oil cooking spray.

Toss the stuffing mix in a bowl with the Butter Buds. Line the bottoms of the casserole dishes with the dressing mixture. Save a cupful for topping.

In a large saucepan, combine the squash and onions with ¼ cup of water. Bring to a boil, stir, cover, and cook 10 to 12 minutes, or until the squash is tender. Turn into a colander and drain well.

Return the squash to the saucepan and add the soup, sour cream, pimentos, and water chestnuts, stirring to mix.

Pour the squash mixture over the dressing and sprinkle with grated cheese, then top with the remainder of the dressing mix. Bake for 30 to 40 minutes, or until browned and bubbling.

Note: If you have trouble finding Butter Buds, use a fat-free pour margarine, such as Fleischmann's.

CRUSTLESS ZUCCHINI QUICHE

2 cups coarsely shredded zucchini
½ cup chopped onion
1 cup egg substitute
1½ cups skim milk
1 tablespoon flour
¼ teaspoon salt
⅛ teaspoon pepper
⅛ teaspoon ground nutmeg
1½ cups shredded fat-free Monterey Jack cheese
1 (4-ounce) can sliced mushrooms, drained

SERVES 6

0 GRAMS FAT

Prep :15
Cook 1:05
Stand :00
Total 1:20

Preheat the oven to 325 degrees.

In a covered saucepan, cook the zucchini and onion in a small amount of water for 5 minutes. Drain well; press out excess liquid.

In a bowl, combine the egg substitute, milk, flour, and seasonings. Stir in the cheese, mushrooms, and zucchini mixture. Pour into an ungreased 10 x 6 x 2-inch baking dish.

On an oven rack, place the baking dish in a larger baking pan. Pour hot water into the larger pan to a depth of 1 inch. Bake at 325 degrees for 1 hour, or until a knife inserted in the center comes out clean.

VEGETABLE SPECIAL

SERVES 4

0.5 GRAM FAT
PER SERVING

Prep :15
Cook :05
Stand :00
Total :20

1 cup sliced yellow squash or any available summer squash
1 small bell pepper, cut into strips
⅓ cup sliced celery
⅓ cup 1-inch-long scallions slices, including tops
½ teaspoon canola oil
1 tablespoon lemon juice
¼ teaspoon lemon pepper
4 ounces Chinese pea pods, fresh, if available, or frozen

Cook the squash, bell pepper, celery, and scallions in oil in a non-stick skillet for about 2 minutes, stirring frequently, until tender-crisp. Stir in the remaining ingredients. Cook about 1 minute longer, until the pea pods are hot.

FRIED CABBAGE

Remember, this looks like a lot, but cabbage cooks down to about half or less.

SERVES 4

0 GRAMS FAT

Prep :10
Cook :10
Stand :00
Total :20

4 to 6 scallions, sliced
1 medium bell pepper, chopped
4 cups chopped cabbage

In a large nonstick skillet sprayed lightly with vegetable oil cooking spray, stir-fry the scallions and pepper for a couple of minutes, just until they begin to soften. Add the cabbage and stir-fry until crisp-tender and lightly browned on the edges.

BUTTERNUT SQUASH

1 butternut squash (about 2 pounds), or other winter squash
½ cup honey
½ cup coconut amaretto
¼ cup packed brown sugar

SERVES 2

0 GRAMS FAT WITHOUT NUTS

Prep :05
Cook :15
Stand :00
Total :20

Pierce the squash several times with a fork and place on a microwave-safe dish. Microwave 4 to 5 minutes on high power, rotating the dish a half-turn after 2 minutes. Cut the squash in quarters lengthwise; discard seeds and membrane. Place squash cut side down in baking dish. Cover with microwave-safe plastic wrap and microwave an additional 4 minutes.

Remove the plastic wrap; drizzle the honey and amaretto over squash. Sprinkle with brown sugar. Replace the plastic wrap, return to the microwave, and cook an additional 2 to 4 minutes, or until very tender.

Serve right in the shell or scoop the pulp out into a serving dish and garnish with a tablespoon of chopped nuts.

BUTTERNUT SQUASH PUDDING

1 butternut squash (about 2 pounds)
1½ cups skim milk
¼ cup packed brown sugar
1 tablespoon cornstarch
¼ teaspoon cinnamon
⅛ teaspoon ground nutmeg
⅛ teaspoon ground allspice
¼ cup egg substitute

SERVES 2

0 GRAMS FAT WITHOUT NUTS AND TOPPING

Prep :05
Cook :22
Stand :45
Total 1:12

Prepare the squash according to the directions above, eliminating the honey, amaretto, and brown sugar. Cook the squash until completely tender; remove plastic wrap. Scoop the pulp into mixing bowl or food processor and measure out 1 cup. Reserve the remaining squash for another purpose. *(continued)*

In a food processor or blender, combine the 1 cup of squash with the skim milk, brown sugar, cornstarch, and spices. Process or mix until smooth. Add the egg substitute and mix until smooth.

Pour into a large microwave-safe bowl; microwave on high 8 to 10 minutes or until thickened, stirring every 2 minutes with a wire whisk. Spoon into individual serving dishes, cover, and chill. Serve with a dollop of light whipped topping and a few sprinkles of chopped nuts.

OVEN-FRIED ONION RINGS

SERVES 4

0 GRAMS FAT

Prep :10
Cook :15
Stand :00
Total :25

1 cup fine dry bread crumbs
2 tablespoons Butter Buds, liquid form (see Note)
Salt and pepper to taste (optional)
½ cup egg substitute or egg whites
2 large onions, sliced ¼ inch thick, separated into rings

Preheat oven to 450 degrees. Lightly spray a large baking sheet with vegetable oil cooking spray.

In a small mixing bowl, combine the bread crumbs and Butter Buds or liquid form margarine, along with the salt and pepper, if using. Mix well. Spread on a sheet of waxed paper on a separate cooking sheet.

Place the egg substitute or whites in a shallow dish. Dip the onion rings in the egg substitute, coating thoroughly, then in the bread crumb mixture. Place the coated onion rings in a single layer on the prepared baking sheet.

Bake for about 15 minutes or until the onions are tender and the coating is crisp and golden.

Note: If you have trouble finding Butter Buds, use a liquid fat-free margarine, such as Fleischmann's.

GREEN TOMATO CASSEROLE

4 white onions
5 green tomatoes
1½ pounds fat-free sharp Cheddar cheese

SERVES 4

0 GRAMS FAT

Prep :15
Cook 1:00
Stand :00
Total 1:15

Preheat the oven to 350 degrees. Lightly spray a 13 x 9-inch glass baking dish with vegetable oil cooking spray.

Slice the onions and tomatoes very thin. Grate the cheese. (I usually buy it already grated.)

Layer tomatoes, onions, and cheese until all are used, ending with the cheese on top.

Bake for about 1 hour, or until the tomatoes and onions are tender.

BREADED OKRA AND TOMATOES

8 cups fresh okra, washed, stemmed, and cut into 1-inch pieces, or frozen sliced
   okra
1 tablespoon vinegar
¾ cup chopped onion
1 small green pepper, sliced into thin rounds
½ teaspoon dried oregano
¼ teaspoon dried basil
¼ teaspoon lemon pepper
2 (8-ounce) cans stewed tomatoes, undrained
½ cup fine dry bread crumbs

SERVES 1

LESS THAN 1
GRAM FAT EN-
TIRE DISH

Prep :15
Cook :40
Stand :00
Total :55

Preheat the oven to 350 degrees. Lightly coat a 9 x 9-inch glass baking dish with vegetable oil cooking spray.

In a large nonaluminum saucepan, cover the okra with water, add the vinegar, and bring to a boil. Cook 2 to 4 minutes, only until crisp-tender. (Adding the vinegar to the okra will keep it from being slimy.) Drain okra in a colander and rinse with warm water. All the slime went down the drain. If using frozen okra, prepare the same way.

Mix the okra, onions, green pepper, oregano, basil, and lemon pepper. Spoon into the prepared baking dish. Pour the tomatoes over, spreading evenly, and top with bread crumbs.

Bake for 30 to 35 minutes, until bubbly.

VEGETABLE-STUFFED PEPPERS

SERVES 2

1 GRAM FAT
PER SERVING

Prep :15
Cook :10
Stand :00
Total :25

½ cup whole-kernel corn, frozen or canned
¼ cup chopped onion
½ cup herbed tomato sauce
⅓ cup quick-cooking rice
Pinch of sugar
Pepper to taste
1 (8-ounce) can chili-flavored beans, drained
1 large bell pepper
1 tablespoon shredded fat-free Cheddar cheese

Combine the corn, onion, and 1 tablespoon of water in a nonstick skillet. Sauté for about 2 minutes; stir in the tomato sauce, un-cooked rice, sugar, and pepper. Cook covered for 2 or 3 minutes or until bubbly, stirring after 1 minute. Stir in beans, cover, and set aside.

Cut the pepper in half lengthwise; remove seeds and mem-branes. Place the pepper cut side down in a microwave-safe dish, cover with plastic wrap, and microwave on high for 3 minutes or until nearly tender. Drain.

Turn the pepper halves cut side up. Fill with the rice mixture, cover, and microwave on high about 2 minutes or until the rice mixture is heated through and the peppers are tender. Sprinkle cheese over peppers before serving.

SLOAN CORN

I hope you don't go to the store and try to find a variety of corn called Sloan corn. This is only a name for sweet corn that my dad tacked onto the corn grown here by my brother and his three children, which is now very well known, statewide.

When my brother's children were about six, eight, and ten years old, he put them in charge of about two acres of sweet corn, in a project to earn money. Now, you already know that the children's dad had to do all the machinery work, planting, and so forth, but he let them manage this project, and sell the corn from the back of the pickup truck under a big shade tree down on the corner, here in Gore. My dad did a good job of training my brother to be a farmer—the corn was big, juicy, tender, and free of worms. (Yes, worms. You have to really spray and watch your corn crops to keep them free of pests such as weevils and worms. Sometimes when you buy corn at a local farm stand or vegetable stand it is just terrible, with worms in the ends of each ear. You might find one or two in an entire bushel of our corn, but more likely you'll find none. They are the largest, prettiest ears of corn imaginable.)

People would be standing in line at daylight waiting for our corn harvest. The corn has to be picked at night while it is cooler so that it will keep better. If you picked it during the hot summer daytime hours, it would cook, from all the heat in the corn and from the sun, in the bottom of the trailer before you got the corn unloaded.

Here in the country we put vegetables in the freezer and can them, for the sake of economy as well as taste. Satisfaction also plays a large part in canning and freezing. I believe I mentioned in an earlier story or book that since Simon & Schuster got hold of me I don't have time to can anymore. My pressure cooker has been retired. I wish you could have seen us putting up corn. We usually did it outside under a tree. We had large lobster-type pots that we heated our water in, over a camp stove or Cajun-style burner. We shucked and washed our corn outside on the patio, and used regular old-fashioned washtubs for this process.

Sometimes we would put up as much as 20 or 30 bushels of corn in one day. The entire family would be out under the tree, shucking, brushing silks, dropping corn into the blanch pot, cooling corn, draining corn; and the big job was cutting it off the ears, bagging it, labeling, carrying to the freezer, and stacking. There is a job for everyone no matter how old or young. If you cut the corn off the cob outdoors, the splatters don't have to be scraped off the walls in the kitchen. (By the time I finish with this story you will really be glad to buy your corn in the supermarket. This is even worse than the potato story, right?)

I want to tell you about the process of harvesting the corn when it is finally ready. They wait until the just-right stage, so you never know what day it will be ready. You can't say, "Well, I think I will can corn on Tuesday." It is sometimes Sunday or Saturday; just depends on Mr. Sunshine. I like to go to the field and pull an ear, shuck it, and eat it right there on the spot, raw. Now, do I like vegetables my brother grows or what??? All the Sloan family loves corn. One way you test the corn to see when it is just-right is to shuck it and pierce a kernel with your fingernail. If it squirts real healthy like, it is ready.

After the corn project started, these two acres they began with grew in popularity and demand until they were raising forty acres at peak project time, and it all had to be picked by hand. You got it—picked by hand. And then they had to pick very early in the morning because they couldn't see to pick at night, of course. They would drive a pickup truck or wagon (pulled by a tractor; it wasn't that long ago) down between two rows with kids on both sides pulling and throwing the ears into the bed of the trailer or truck. It looked like it was raining corn because they would pick two or three rows at a time on each side of the truck. These three kids did *not* do all this picking themselves. They proceeded to hire other young people in our small town who wanted to make some extra summer money, as most kids do. My niece and nephews would buy cases of pop and boxes of candy bars to give their workers a break. I thought that was nice.

They would walk up and down the length of these fields until the entire crop was harvested—not in one day by any means; this would go on for several days until the corn was all picked. But they did have to concentrate on doing a pretty large area at a time or per day, because once corn is ready and stays in the field for a few days the kernels start to get hard. When this happens it means you have lost your crop—no one wants corn that is tough and hard.

When the demand got so large, my brother invested in a one-row corn picker. This machine is pulled by a tractor and has a trailer following the picker. The picker has a chute on the back where the corn is ejected after it has been picked from the stalks. Several kids ride back there and cull out the little nubbins and stalks that slip through the machine. They have a big floodlight hooked onto the machine. Remember, this all takes place from first dark in the evening to daybreak the next morning.

There are peddlers who bring their trucks, trailers, wagons, or whatever they are hauling their corn in, and park them at the end of the field and sometime during the night the Corn Fairy fills up their carrier. Really what happens is there are big pitchfork-type shovels that transfer the corn onto the peddlers' vehicles. Yes, they still buy pop and candy for their midnight treats. Do you suppose I could talk those young teenagers into eating fat-free candy and diet pop? *Not!*

My dad always loved corn cooked any way you would cook it. We would put up several dozen ears on the cob for the big visits and cookouts involving the aunts, as told in the first book. Dad would always say, "Must be Sloan corn!" I don't care if it was Jolly Green Giant, cream style, or whatever, he would say that anyway—but he always knew what was really Sloan corn. We rarely had anything else on any of our tables. I still serve it, but without the butter.

Corn is almost always ready on or near the Fourth of July in this part of the country. We could count on having to do corn on the Fourth about nine times out of ten. There is still the farm stand on the corner, and many people who come to the lake (we live just below Lake Tenkiler here in Oklahoma) have been buying corn from these kids for thirty years. The three kids, who are now adults, also have sideline occupations other than their corn adventure, but it will carry on. Their occupations? One is a doctor, one is a school-teacher, and the third—you guessed it—is a farmer. He was the one who always would "ramrod" the corn adventures.

Corn played a welcome part in the education of all three corn entrepreneurs. As I write this, it is late March and the tractors are rolling—preparations are under way for corn planting. Fourth of July will be here in a short while.

I bet you have something in your family that is as special as corn is to the Sloan family.

CORN ON THE COB

To boil: Husk the corn, remove the silk, and place the corn in a large pot of boiling water. Return to a boil and cook about 4 or 5 minutes, or until tender.

To microwave: Clean the corn as described above, wrap each ear in plastic wrap, leaving one end open to let steam escape, and microwave each ear about 3 to 4 minutes, until kernels are tender. Holding the corn with tongs or a towel, remove the plastic wrap. Be careful not to burn yourself with the steam.

To blanch corn: Have a large container of water boiling over high heat. Very carefully, drop the corn into the boiling water and permit it to stand for 1 minute. Remove and plunge into ice water until chilled through. Remember to leave in the water long enough to chill the cob too. Remove from the water and drain. Use as desired.

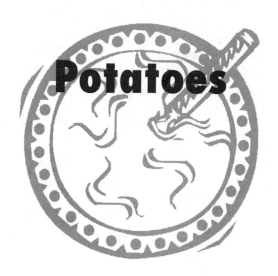

Potatoes

MASHED POTATOES

SERVES 6

**1 GRAM FAT
ENTIRE DISH**

**Prep :20
Cook :30
Stand :00
Total :50**

6 to 8 medium potatoes
¾ cup buttermilk (skim or 1 gram fat per cup)
Salt and pepper to taste
2 teaspoons Butter Buds sprinkles, or ¼ cup liquid form

Peel and cube the potatoes into about 2-inch squares. Place the potatoes in a large saucepan and cover with 2 quarts of cold water (add more if needed to cover). Bring to a boil, lower the heat to medium, and slow-boil until tender, about 30 minutes. Drain, reserving about ¾ cup liquid.

Transfer the potatoes to a medium glass mixing bowl. Using a hand-held electric mixer, crush the potatoes with the mixer beaters up and down a little before you turn the mixer on, to get rid of lumps. Start the mixer and start mashing the potatoes. When about half mashed, start adding buttermilk, seasonings, and Butter Buds. Add a little of the liquid reserved from boiling to get them to the right fluffy consistency. Turn the mixer on high and very vigorously move the mixer in circles around the edge of the bowl as you continue to mix. This will fluff your potatoes. Serve hot.

Variation: Instead of buttermilk, use just plain skim milk and Butter Buds. If you use skim milk, it is nice to heat the milk; this will keep the potatoes hot longer.

MASHED POTATO CASSEROLE

2 pounds baking potatoes
1 (8-ounce) package fat-free cream cheese, at room temperature
1 cup plain nonfat yogurt
½ teaspoon garlic powder
¼ teaspoon salt
2 tablespoons Butter Buds, liquid form
½ teaspoon paprika

SERVES 6

0 GRAMS FAT

Prep :20
Cook :60
Stand :00
Total 1:20

Peel the potatoes and cut into 2-inch chunks. Place in a large saucepan, cover with cold water, and bring to a boil. Lower the heat to medium and continue to cook until very tender, about 30 minutes.

Meanwhile, preheat the oven to 350 degrees. Lightly coat an 11 x 7-inch baking dish with vegetable oil cooking spray.

Drain the potatoes and put in a mixing bowl. Add the cream cheese, yogurt, garlic powder, and salt. Beat at medium speed with an electric mixer until smooth.

Spoon into the prepared baking dish, drizzle with Butter Buds, and sprinkle with paprika. Bake uncovered for 30 minutes.

SPINACH STORY

My dad was a farmer and my brother and my nephew are farmers. That's right—I am a farmer's daughter. Spinach holds a special fondness in my memories. As well as being one of my favorite vegetables, it is very good for you. It is full of iron and vitamins and is a good cancer-fighting source. Besides, it makes you strong like Popeye.

During World War II my dad went down to the county courthouse to sign up to serve his country. I can remember the day so clearly. My mom, brother, and I sat on the lawn of the courthouse while he went in to take care of business. We were very sad. When he came out, he had wonderful news. The Army wanted him to raise spinach for them, so we would get to keep dad at home with us while he was serving his country. That was the beginning of the Spinach Impact in the Sloan family.

Dad planted large fields of spinach. When it was to be harvested, in those days, it had to be cut by hand. I am talking about getting down on your knees with a large sharp knife, holding the bunch of spinach (it grew in small bunches right on the ground) in one hand and cutting with the other. This very often resulted in cut fingers, sometimes serious cuts. You then put your spinach in a wooden bushel basket. They must have weighed 30 pounds per basket. You packed and smashed it down. Then you carried the basket to the truck where there was a scale you put it on to be weighed. If it didn't weigh what it was supposed to, you took it back and cut some more. You got paid 10 cents a basket. That was my job: I got to hand out the dimes. I was of course supervised by an adult, as I was only about six years old. The baskets of spinach were then thrown up onto the truck, dumped out, and tromped down. Dad then had to haul it to a town about 55 miles away. It was late in the day and sometimes night before he would return.

If he had a good crop he would sometimes buy us a little present before returning. One time I got a little red ring, my first ring. I was so proud of it, I thought I had a 3-carat diamond, but I dropped it in the chicken yard and my pet chicken ate it before I could grab it. Oh, well. Was great while it lasted. My chicken's name was Carter Red.

My brother and nephew now raise spinach, but it is much different in this day and time. They have large equipment and improved hybrid seed that stands up higher off the ground and is much larger. It is quite a treat to go watch the "cutting of the spinach" and remember how it used to be. I had a picture of the old truck in my dad's field with my grandfather sitting on the running board. I had it enlarged and gave it to my brother.

They still dump the spinach into the trucks, but it is a semi truck that drives alongside the cutting machine, which is pulled by a huge tractor. They talk by remote phones to each other to stay in line. Then there are the trompers. Yes, they still tromp it to pack it down in order to get more on the truck. As you see, it is very light, and without tromping it you would have very little weight when you got to the canners. It is sold by the pound just as we buy it in the grocery stores.

My brother raises spinach for a company named—you guessed it—"Popeye" spinach. We always enjoy going over to the field, just standing and looking out across the beautiful green waves of luscious vegetation and of course filching a bit for the freezer. I also like to use spinach leaves on sandwiches instead of lettuce. It is wonderful.

You can see from the short story that spinach is very special to our family.

SPINACH POTATO CASSEROLE

SERVES 6

0 GRAMS FAT

Prep :20
Cook :50
Stand :00
Total 1:10

6 to 8 potatoes
1 cup fat-free sour cream
1/4 cup fat-free margarine, at room temperature
2 teaspoons salt
1/4 teaspoon pepper
1/3 cup chopped scallions, tops and all
1 (10-ounce) package frozen chopped spinach, thawed and squeezed dry
1 cup shredded fat-free Cheddar cheese

Peel and cube the potatoes, place in a medium-size saucepan, and cover with water. Boil until tender, 20 to 30 minutes.

While the potatoes are boiling, preheat the oven to 400 degrees. Lightly spray a 2-quart casserole with vegetable oil cooking spray.

Drain the potatoes, place in a large bowl, and crush, then mash, with a hand-held electric mixer. Beat in the sour cream, margarine, salt, and pepper. Add the scallions and spinach and stir until thoroughly mixed.

Spoon into the prepared casserole and bake uncovered for 15 minutes. Spread the shredded cheese evenly over the casserole and bake 5 or 6 minutes longer, or until the cheese is melted.

CORN AND POTATO CASSEROLE

1 medium onion, chopped
¼ cup chopped green pepper
1 (32-ounce) package fat-free frozen hash brown potatoes
2 cups frozen whole corn kernels
1 (16-ounce) container fat-free sour cream
1 (10¾-ounce) can Healthy Request cream of celery soup
1 cup shredded fat-free Cheddar cheese
2 cups cornflake crumbs

SERVES 6

4.75 GRAMS
FAT ENTIRE
DISH

Prep :10
Cook 1:05
Stand :00
Total 1:15

Preheat the oven to 350 degrees. Spray an 11 x 7-inch baking dish lightly with vegetable oil cooking spray.

In a nonstick skillet, sauté the onion and green pepper in a couple of tablespoons of water until tender, about 5 minutes

Combine the hash brown potatoes, corn, onion and pepper, sour cream, soup, and cheese in a large bowl. Stir well. Spoon into the prepared baking dish and top with cornflake crumbs.

Bake uncovered for 1 hour or until golden brown.

Note: If making ahead, after assembling in the baking dish, cover with plastic wrap and store in the refrigerator. Set out at room temperature about 15 minutes before baking time. Do not add cornflake crumbs until baking time.

OVEN-FRIED SWEET POTATOES

SERVES 4

SLIGHT TRACE
OF FAT PER
SERVING

Prep :15
Cook :40
Stand :00
Total :55

3 large sweet potatoes
½ cup skim milk
¾ to 1 cup fine, dry bread crumbs

Preheat the oven to 350 degrees. Lightly spray a baking sheet with vegetable oil cooking spray.

Scrub the potatoes, but do not peel. Cut them crosswise into the thickness you desire. Dip in skim milk and coat with bread crumbs. Place the sweet potato slices on the prepared baking sheet and spray the top of each piece lightly with cooking spray.

Bake uncovered for 15 to 20 minutes. Turn the potatoes and bake 15 to 20 minutes more, depending on the thickness, until tender.

SWEET POTATO FLUFF

SERVES 6

0 GRAMS FAT

Prep :15
Cook :20
Stand :00
Total :35

3 medium sweet potatoes
2 tablespoons orange juice
1⅓ teaspoons cinnamon
½ cup packed brown sugar
¼ cup coconut amaretto

Peel the potatoes and cut them into 2-inch chunks. Place them in a medium saucepan, cover with water, and boil gently until tender, about 15 to 20 minutes.

Drain the potatoes and put in a mixing bowl. Add the orange juice, cinnamon, brown sugar, and half the amaretto. With an electric mixer, beat the potatoes until fluffy, adding amaretto as needed. You may need just a little more than ¼ cup, especially after you taste it.

SWEET POTATOES

3 medium sweet potatoes
2 tablespoons orange juice
½ cup honey
¼ cup packed brown sugar
¾ cup coconut amaretto

SERVES 4

0 GRAMS FAT

Prep :10
Cook :50
Stand :00
Total 1:00

Preheat the oven to 350 degrees. Lightly spray a 3-quart baking dish with vegetable oil cooking spray.

Peel the sweet potatoes and cut into 1½-inch chunks. Place in the prepared baking dish. Sprinkle orange juice over evenly. Stream honey evenly over all, sprinkle brown sugar over the honey, and pour amaretto over evenly. Really doesn't matter how you pour these four ingredients over these potatoes, they are going to be so good.

Bake uncovered for 45 to 50 minutes or until tender and bubbly.

Tip: If you are in a hurry you can boil the potatoes until they start to get tender. Peel and cube them, place in the baking dish, and continue with the directions.

SWEET POTATO CRISP

Make ahead for the holidays.

SERVES 16

0 GRAMS FAT
(NUTS OMIT-
TED)

Prep :35
Cook 1:20
Stand :00
Total 1:55

3½ pounds medium sweet potatoes
⅓ cup packed brown sugar
⅓ cup orange juice
½ cup egg substitute
3 tablespoons Kahlúa
1½ teaspoons pumpkin pie spice
1 tablespoon Butter Buds, liquid form

Topping:
¼ cup finely chopped pecans, toasted
3 tablespoons all-purpose or whole-wheat flour
¼ cup packed brown sugar
1 teaspoon ground cinnamon
1 tablespoon Butter Buds, liquid form

Wash the potatoes, place in a deep stockpot, cover with water, and cook 35 to 40 minutes, or until tender. Drain and cool. When cool enough to handle, peel potatoes and place in a large mixing bowl. Mash until smooth.

Preheat the oven to 350 degrees. Lightly spray a 2-quart baking dish with vegetable oil cooking spray.

Stir the ⅓ cup brown sugar, orange juice, egg substitute, Kahlúa, pie spice, and Butter Buds into the mashed sweet potatoes. Transfer to the prepared baking dish.

Make the topping: Combine the pecans, flour, ¼ cup brown sugar, cinnamon, and 1 tablespoon Butter Buds in a small bowl and mix with a fork. Sprinkle over the sweet potatoes. Bake uncovered for 40 minutes.

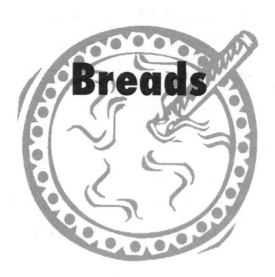

Breads

"CORNMEAL MANIA"

I know you can buy cornmeal in the store for a very low price, but let me tell you how I come by my cornmeal.

First you have to harvest the ears of corn, usually the last of August in about 100-degree weather. You guessed it—filching off brother again. He grows both sweet and field corn, and for cornmeal we use field corn.

The stalks are usually about 8 to 9 feet tall. Now, I am only 5′3″, so I am talking away above my head. (Bob is 6′4″ and I am still talking way above.)

Let me set the mood here for you. It is August, 100 degrees, stalks 9 feet tall and about 30 inches apart, which means they are touching stalk leaves all along the way. The leaves are flat and thin and sharp on the edge, so you have to be real careful or they will give you a paperlike cut if you brush through them too fast.

Have I got your attention, and are you really feeling like you would love to go out and pick some corn? Here we go! We have five-gallon buckets. The corn is dry so it is pretty easy to pick, but you also have to shuck it and the shucks are hard to get off, because they aren't dry enough to turn loose easy. When your bucket is full, pack it back to the (you thought for sure I was going to say *wagon*) truck. Hot deluxe by now. We always take towels to dry up the—down here in Oklahoma we call it sweat—and ice water to drink. Of course you know the more you drink the more you . . . Yep, down in the corn row I go. Carter Red should see me now.

Get our corn home and we have to store it for several weeks until it gets really dry. Then we have to prepare it for going to the cornmill. You nub your corn; that is, hit it on the concrete floor or a rock to knock off any bad kernels on the very tip end. Then we have a corn sheller that was my grandfather's; you just drop your ear of corn in, turn the handle, and it shells the corn and spits out the cob on the side. It just tickles me to death to watch it work. I love it. There is a wooden box that the sheller sits on and the kernels drop into it. When finished shelling you then have to clean the corn.

We do this cleaning job by setting up an electric fan—yes, we do have electricity—then we pour the corn from one container to another in front of the fan; it blows out all the husk and silks. After about four passes by the fan the corn is clean enough to go to the mill.

Going to the mill is always a treat for Bob and me. It is about a forty-minute drive and way out in the country. The man who has this operation has updated and modernized somewhat. He has an electric mill, powered by a tractor that has a big pulley belt hooked up to it. It is loud and the meal dust is flying. We look like we have been in a cornmeal dust storm when it is finished. But it is too good to not stand right there and watch. The meal is hot when it is put into the containers, usually brown paper bags. It costs us five cents a pound to have it ground. Is that great or what?

The meal is a little heavier than store bought and a wonderful yellow color. It is absolutely the best thing ever to coat fish with. We bag up meal and give it for Christmas gifts. All our city friends love it, and so do our country friends.

The mill owner has sweet potatoes and apples that he grows, harvests, and sells in the fall. A trip to the mill is always one of my favorite fall activities. Makes you forget about that hot harvest. This meal sure makes good cornbread too. It is a little heavier than that made from the store-bought meal. I love it. I don't slow down long enough to make it very much anymore. But I do make it fat-free now.

TEX-MEX MUFFINS

MAKES
ABOUT 18
MUFFINS,
2
MUFFINS
PER SERV-
ING

ONLY A SLIGHT
TRACE OF FAT
PER MUFFIN

Prep :10
Cook :30
Stand :00
Total :40

1½ cups yellow cornmeal
1 teaspoon baking soda
½ teaspoon salt
1 (2-ounce) jar diced pimentos, drained
1 cup shredded fat-free Cheddar cheese
½ cup finely chopped onion
¼ cup chopped green chiles, undrained
½ cup egg substitute
1 cup skim milk
1 (8-ounce) can yellow cream-style corn

Preheat the oven to 400 degrees. Lightly spray two muffin pans with vegetable oil cooking spray.

In a mixing bowl, combine the cornmeal, baking soda, and salt; stir in the pimentos, cheese, onion, and chiles. Make a well in the center. Combine the egg substitute, milk, and corn; add to the dry ingredients, stirring just until moistened. Spoon into the prepared muffin pans, filling the cups ¾ full. Bake for 30 minutes or until golden. Remove from the pans immediately.

Variation: Add 1 teaspoon jalapeño peppers, chopped fine, for a spicier Mexican flavor.

BUTTERMILK CORN BREAD

1½ cups cornmeal
¾ cup all-purpose flour
1 teaspoon baking powder
½ teaspoon salt
1 teaspoon baking soda
½ cup egg substitute
1 cup skim buttermilk (1 gram fat per cup)
1 tablespoon canola oil

SERVES 8

1 GRAM FAT
PER SERVING

Prep :20
Cook :35
Stand :00
Total :55

Preheat the oven to 400 degrees. Lightly spray a 9 x 9-inch baking pan with vegetable oil cooking spray. Or preheat a medium-size cast-iron skillet in the oven; then coat with cooking spray just before adding the batter.

In a mixing bowl, combine the cornmeal, flour, baking powder, salt, and baking soda. Stir to mix all ingredients. Make a well in the middle; add the egg substitute, buttermilk, and oil. Stir these three ingredients and gradually start mixing the meal mixture into the buttermilk mixture. You may need to add a little water; stir in about 2 tablespoons at a time until all the dry ingredients are moistened.

Turn the batter into the prepared pan and bake for 35 to 45 minutes, or until the corn bread is lightly browned and springy to the touch.

PICANTE CORN BREAD

SERVES 8

0 GRAMS FAT

Prep :10
Cook :40
Stand :00
Total :50

2 cups fat-free self-rising cornmeal mix
½ cup egg substitute
1 cup skim milk
⅓ cup picante sauce

Preheat the oven to 400 degrees. Lightly spray an 8 x 8-inch baking pan or medium cast-iron skillet with vegetable oil cooking spray.

Mix the cornmeal, egg substitute, and milk. When thoroughly moistened, add the picante sauce. Continue mixing, adding a little water if necessary, to get a medium heavy batter.

Pour the batter into the prepared pan and bake for about 35 to 40 minutes, or until done to the touch in the middle and golden brown on top.

MEXICAN CORN BREAD

SERVES 8

0.05 GRAM FAT
PER 4-INCH-
SQUARE
SERVING

Prep :10
Cook :40
Stand :00
Total :50

2 cups fat-free self-rising cornmeal mix
1½ cups skim milk
½ cup egg substitute
½ cup whole-kernel corn
¼ cup finely chopped onion
¼ cup finely chopped pimento
6 jalapeño pepper rings, chopped fine

Preheat the oven to 400 degrees. Lightly coat a 9 x 9-inch baking pan with vegetable oil cooking spray.

In a medium-size mixing bowl, mix all of the above ingredients. You may need to add a little water or a little more milk to get the consistency you desire. Pour into the prepared pan and smooth out level. Bake for about 30 to 40 minutes or until lightly browned.

Variation: Fried Mexican Corn Bread: This batter may be cooked like pancakes. I call it dry-fry. This is a good way to fix corn bread in the summer without heating up your kitchen and also a way to cook in a hurry. Just use a nonstick skillet and spray it lightly with cooking spray. Spoon in batter just as you would a pancake, about ¼ cup to a cake. Turn when bubbles appear on the surface and cook on the flip side until brown. Ummm, good!!!

CRANBERRY NUT BREAD

3 cups all-purpose flour
1 cup sugar
1 tablespoon baking powder
¼ teaspoon baking soda
¼ teaspoon salt (optional)
¼ cup egg substitute
1⅔ cups skim milk
¼ cup applesauce
2 teaspoons finely shredded orange zest
1 cup coarsely chopped cranberries
¼ cup chopped English walnuts or pecans
Powdered Sugar Glaze (see next page) (optional)

MAKES 1 LARGE OR 2 SMALL LOAVES; SERVES 4

2 GRAMS FAT PER SERVING

Prep :20
Cook 1:15
Stand :10
Total 1:45

Preheat the oven to 350 degrees. Lightly spray one 9 x 5 x 3-inch loaf pan or two 7½ x 3½ x 2-inch loaf pans with vegetable oil cooking spray.

Stir together in a large mixing bowl the flour, sugar, baking powder, baking soda, and salt, if desired. In a smaller mixing bowl, stir together the egg substitute, milk, applesauce, and orange zest. Add to the flour mixture, stirring just until combined. Stir in the cranberries and walnuts. Pour the batter into the prepared pans.

Bake for 1 to 1¼ hours for the 9-inch pan, 45 minutes for the 7-inch pans, or until a toothpick inserted near the center comes out clean. *(continued)*

Cool the bread in the pan on a wire rack for 10 minutes. Remove the bread from the pan and cool completely on the rack. Wrap and store overnight for the best slicing consistency. Drizzle with Powdered Sugar Glaze if desired.

POWDERED SUGAR GLAZE

0 GRAMS FAT

Prep :05
Cook :00
Stand :00
Total :05

1½ cups powdered sugar
½ teaspoon vanilla extract
2 tablespoons skim milk

Mix all above ingredients together until smooth. If necessary, add more or less milk, to get the consistency desired.

YEASTED PUMPKIN OR SQUASH BREAD

MAKES 1
LOAF

0 GRAMS FAT

Prep :15
Cook :40
Stand 2:15
Total 3:10

2 tablespoons Butter Buds, liquid form
1 envelope (¼ ounce) active dry yeast
⅓ cup warm water
2 tablespoons packed light brown sugar
¼ cup egg substitute
1 teaspoon grated orange zest
½ teaspoon ground cinnamon
¼ teaspoon salt
⅛ teaspoon ground cloves
½ cup mashed cooked pumpkin, or acorn or butternut squash
2¾ cups all-purpose flour
1 large egg white, lightly beaten

Lightly coat a 9 x 5 x 3-inch loaf pan with vegetable oil cooking spray.

Set Butter Buds out of the refrigerator to warm to room temperature.

Rinse a large mixing bowl with hot water to take the chill off; dry well. In this bowl, combine the yeast, water, and 1 tablespoon of sugar. Let stand about 5 minutes or until bubbly; stir until yeast is dissolved. To the yeast mixture, add the egg substitute, orange zest, cinnamon, salt, cloves, and pumpkin or squash, along with the Butter Buds. Stir until thoroughly mixed. Add the flour, 1 cup at a time, to make a firm but not dry dough.

Turn the dough out onto a floured surface and knead vigorously for 6 to 8 minutes. Coat a large bowl with cooking spray, shape the dough into a ball, place in the bowl, and turn so that the dough is coated on all sides. Cover with a clean dish towel and let rise in a warm draft-free place until doubled in bulk, about 1½ hours.

Punch down the dough, knead for 1 or 2 minutes, shape into a loaf, and place in the prepared pan, seam side down. Cover with the towel and let the loaf rise to 1 inch above the rim of the pan, about 45 minutes. Shortly before the end of rising time, preheat the oven to 375 degrees.

Brush the top of the loaf with the egg white and bake for 35 to 40 minutes or until the top is golden and the loaf sounds hollow when tapped.

Variation: Drizzle with a sugar glaze or serve plain. The bread can be made when squash or pumpkins are in season and frozen for the holidays. Makes a great gift also: wrap in a pretty colored plastic wrap and tie a bow around the loaf.

Cakes, Pies, and Cookies

A GOOD FRIEND CAKE

SERVES
EVERYONE

0 GRAMS FAT

Prep: many
hours
Cook: cen-
turies
Total: lifetime

1 cup Kindness
2 cups Courtesy
3 cups Truthfulness
2½ cups Dependability
1 cup Freedom
2 tablespoons Industry
4 cups Obedience
1½ cups Honesty
2 cups Modesty
3 cups Sharing
6½ cups Honor to Parents

Simmer all ingredients over a gentle fire of family love, for a lifetime. Serve with smiles and heartfelt praise and good humor.

APPLICIOUS CARAMEL CAKE

SERVES 12

8 GRAMS FAT
ENTIRE CAKE
(WITHOUT
NUTS)

Prep :20
Cook :45
Stand :00
Total 1:05

1 (18-ounce) package caramel-flavor cake mix
1 (1-ounce) package sugar free butterscotch instant pudding mix
¾ cup egg substitute
¾ cup applesauce
⅓ cup fat-free mayonnaise or salad dressing, such as Miracle Whip
2 Granny Smith apples
1 cup packed brown sugar
½ cup chopped nuts (optional)
Fat-free margarine spray (has a pump-type spray on top)

Preheat the oven to 350 degrees. Lightly spray a 13 x 9-inch baking dish with vegetable oil cooking spray.

In a large mixing bowl, combine the cake mix, pudding mix, egg substitute, applesauce, mayonnaise, and ⅓ cup of water. Mix well. Pour the batter into prepared baking dish.

Peel and thinly slice the apples (up and down to make half-moon slices). Place on top of the batter, forming three lengthwise rows. Press the apple slices slightly down into the batter.

In a small bowl, combine the brown sugar and nuts if using. Mix and sprinkle over the apples. Spray the topping with margarine until it looks damp.

Bake at 350 degrees for 40 to 45 minutes, or until a toothpick inserted near the center comes out clean. Cool on a rack and serve from pan.

Variations: Serve with fat-free vanilla yogurt or ice cream. Drizzle caramel (fat-free) ice cream topping over all.

CARROT CAKE

SERVES 12

1 GRAM FAT
PER SERVING
(WITHOUT
NUTS)

Prep :15
Cook :40
Stand :00
Total :55

1¼ cups pitted prunes, halved
½ cup hot water
2 cups all-purpose flour
2 teaspoons ground cinnamon
1½ teaspoons baking soda
½ teaspoon salt
4 cups shredded carrots
2 cups sugar
½ cup pineapple juice
½ cup egg substitute
2 teaspoons vanilla extract
Cream Cheese Frosting (see next page) (optional)
½ cup chopped pecans (optional)

Preheat the oven to 350 degrees. Coat a 9 x 13-inch baking pan with vegetable oil cooking spray.

Combine the prunes and hot water in a food processor or blender container. Process or blend until finely chopped, scraping down sides occasionally. Set aside.

In a medium mixing bowl, combine the flour, cinnamon, baking soda, and salt. Set aside.

In a large bowl, mix prune purée, carrots, sugar, juice, egg substitute, and vanilla. Add the flour mixture, stirring well until blended. Pour into the prepared pan.

Bake at 350 degrees for 30 to 40 minutes or until a toothpick inserted near the center comes out clean. Cool on a wire rack, dust with powdered sugar or cover with frosting (recipe below).

Cream Cheese Frosting

1¾ cups powdered sugar
1 (8-ounce) package fat-free cream cheese, at room temperature
1 teaspoon vanilla extract

Very carefully mix the above ingredients with a wire whisk, only until blended. (Fat-free cream cheese will break down if overmixed.) Spread on the cake. Sprinkle chopped pecans over if desired (will add more fat grams).

STRAWBERRY SUNDAE CAKE

SERVES 12

1.5 GRAMS FAT
PER SERVING

Prep :15
Cook :45
Stand :00
Total 1:00

1 (18-ounce) package strawberry cake mix
1 (3-ounce) package strawberry gelatin dessert mix (fat-free, sugar-free)
1 (10-ounce) package frozen strawberries, thawed (reserve ¼ cup juice for frosting)
½ cup applesauce
¾ cup egg substitute
¼ cup chopped pecans (optional)
Strawberry Frosting (see below)

Preheat the oven to 350 degrees. Spray a 9 x 13-inch baking dish with vegetable oil cooking spray.

In a large mixing bowl, combine the dry cake mix, gelatin dessert mix, strawberries, applesauce, and egg substitute. With an electric mixer, mix well. Stir in pecans if desired, reserving a few for the topping.

Pour the batter into the prepared baking dish. Bake for 40 to 45 minutes, or until a toothpick inserted near the center comes out clean. Cool on a wire rack until slightly warm. Spread with Strawberry Frosting. Top with pecans if desired.

Strawberry Frosting

2 cups powdered sugar
2 teaspoons fat-free margarine, at room temperature
¼ teaspoon vanilla extract
3 to 4 tablespoons strawberry juice (reserved from Strawberry Sundae Cake)

0 GRAMS FAT

Prep :05
Cook :00
Stand :00
Total :05

Combine the powdered sugar, margarine, and vanilla. Add strawberry juice a tablespoon at a time until frosting is desired consistency.

LEMON BUNDT CAKE

1 (18-ounce) package lemon cake mix
¾ cup egg substitute
⅔ cup fat-free mayonnaise (such as Miracle Whip)
⅔ cup applesauce
1 tablespoon lemon juice

SERVES 12

3.5 GRAMS FAT
ENTIRE CAKE

Prep :15
Cook :55
Stand :10
Total 1:20

Preheat the oven to 350 degrees. Spray a medium-size Bundt pan with vegetable oil cooking spray.

In a large mixing bowl, combine the cake mix, egg substitute, mayonnaise, applesauce, lemon juice, and ¼ cup of water. Mix 3 to 4 minutes with a hand-held electric mixer until well blended and smooth.

Pour the batter into the prepared pan. Bake for 50 to 55 minutes, or until a toothpick inserted near the center of the cake comes out clean. Cool in the pan on a wire rack for 10 minutes. Remove from the pan and cool completely on the rack.

APPLE CAKE

SERVES 8

1 GRAM FAT
PER SERVING
(WITHOUT
NUTS)

Prep :20
Cook :40
Stand :00
Total 1:00

1 cup sugar
¼ cup applesauce
¼ cup egg substitute
1 cup all-purpose flour
1 teaspoon baking soda
½ teaspoon ground cinnamon
¼ teaspoon salt (optional)
2 cups shredded peeled tart apples
¼ cup chopped walnuts (optional)
Vanilla Sauce (opposite page)

Preheat the oven to 350 degrees. Spray an 8 x 8-inch baking pan with vegetable oil cooking spray.

In a mixing bowl, stir together the sugar and applesauce. Add the egg substitute and mix well. In a separate bowl, mix the flour, baking soda, cinnamon, and salt, if using. Beat together the wet ingredients and the flour mixture just until smooth. Fold in the apples and walnuts, if desired.

Spread the batter in the prepared baking dish. Bake for 35 to 40 minutes, or until the cake shrinks slightly from the sides of the pan and is springy to the touch. Remove to a rack and cool slightly in the pan. Serve the warm cake with warm Vanilla Sauce. (opposite page).

VANILLA SAUCE

1 cup sugar
2 tablespoons cornstarch
½ cup evaporated skim milk
½ cup Butter Buds, liquid form (see Note)
1½ teaspoons vanilla extract

VERY LOW-FAT

Prep :03
Cook :02
Stand :00
Total :05

Combine the sugar, cornstarch, and milk in a saucepan. Bring to a boil over medium heat; boil for 2 minutes. Remove from heat and add Butter Buds or margarine and vanilla. Stir to blend. Serve warm.

Note: If you have trouble finding liquid Butter Buds, use liquid fat-free margarine, such as Fleischmann's.

POPPY SEED BUNDT CAKE

1 (18-ounce) package light yellow cake mix, 97% fat-free
½ cup sugar
⅓ cup canola oil
1 cup plain nonfat yogurt
1 cup egg substitute
2 tablespoons lemon juice
2 tablespoons poppy seeds
Lemon Glaze (see below)

SERVES 12

4 GRAMS FAT
PER SERVING

Prep :20
Cook :40
Stand :10
Total 1:10

Preheat the oven to 350 degrees. Coat a medium-size Bundt pan with vegetable oil cooking spray.

Combine the cake mix and sugar in a large mixing bowl. Add the oil, yogurt, egg substitute, lemon juice, and ¼ cup of water. Beat at medium speed with an electric mixer 6 minutes. Stir in the poppy seeds.

Pour the batter into the prepared pan. Bake for 40 minutes or until a toothpick comes out clean from the center area of the cake.

(continued)

Cool in the pan on a wire rack for 10 minutes. Remove from pan. Drizzle with lemon glaze. Cool completely on the wire rack.

Lemon Glaze

1 cup powdered sugar
2 tablespoons lemon juice (you may want to add more for desired consistency)

Combine these ingredients and stir until smooth.

PUMPKIN PATCH STORY

As you already know, my brother is a farmer. He raises many things, according to what the market is asking for. He has a big pumpkin patch almost every year alongside one of his regular crops. He has four grandchildren, and I think that the pumpkin patch is more for pleasure than profit. He should know by now that I am the biggest kid in the family and I have more enjoyment out of these types of things than anyone else on the farm.

I just love driving down the road and all of a sudden there are all these orange balls in all sizes, all shapes, and all colors. I used to think that all pumpkins were orange. Not so. He has orange, orange with green specks, orange with green streaks, yellow, white, light green, dark green, and the shapes are numerous. I was amazed the first year I got to really walk out into a pumpkin patch and choose my very own pumpkin. If you think that was an easy job, think again.

I have this most wonderful husband in the world; he has patience untold. I would say, "This one, it's the prettiest and the biggest." He would carry it to the truck. I would walk around a little longer and guess what, I found this *really* perfect one this time. "Honey, over here! Please, just this one more." The truck is starting to lean from the weight on one side. He would come get that perfect one, and meanwhile I am wandering around: "Honey." "Honey." "Honey."

I could have fed the U.S. Army pumpkin pie from that one trip. I wound up having to take some back and giving some to our children who live in the city, to decorate their yards with. But it was really fun.

In this big pumpkin patch were planted some ornamental gourds, tiny ones that looked just like miniature pumpkins, in great colors, and some really unusual shapes to say the least. Of course I had the same problem choosing as I did with the big pumpkins. This wasn't quite so hard on my poor husband, as the pumpkins might weigh as much as 30 or 40 pounds. These weigh ounces. I just needed a larger bucket to put those darling little gourds in. I had all kinds of lovely fall and holiday arrangements, all over the house, on the porch, everywhere. As you have probably guessed by now, if you have my first book and have read this book, I do like to filch off my brother's wonderful, beautiful crops. Bob and I say that you can't be much closer to God than over in the bottom in one of those large fields of swaying greens on a cool breezy morning. It is indescribably serene.

I have a granddaughter named Tracy. She has show-and-tell in school, as most children do. I also have a white car. One day I took Tracy over to the pumpkin patch to gather a couple pumpkins for Halloween. She wanted to take them to school for show-and-tell. The teacher told her mother Tracy was talking about the trip, explaining all about the goings on, when she hesitated and said, "My grandma just drove that big ol' white car right down the middle of that pumpkin patch," and giggled. That is a special memory for both of us. (We really did drive right down the middle, stopping now and then to pick just the perfect one. I also took pictures of her sitting on some of the really big ones.) I hope that every time Tracy sees a pumpkin and/or eats a pumpkin dessert she will think of her grandma.

PUMPKIN CAKE

2¾ cups all-purpose flour
1 teaspoon baking soda
½ teaspoon baking powder
¼ teaspoon salt
1 teaspoon ground nutmeg
1 teaspoon ground cloves
1 teaspoon cinnamon
¾ cup egg substitute
1¾ cups granulated sugar
1 cup applesauce
1 (16-ounce) can pumpkin
1 cup raisins, chopped (optional)
½ cup chopped pecans (optional)

Glaze:
1½ cups powdered sugar
2 to 3 teaspoons skim milk

SERVES 16

0 GRAMS FAT
(IF PECANS
OMITTED)

Prep :25
Cook 1:15
Stand :10
Total 1:50

Preheat the oven to 350 degrees. Spray a 12-cup Bundt pan or a 10-inch tube pan with vegetable oil cooking spray.

In a large mixing bowl, combine the flour, baking soda, baking powder, salt, nutmeg, cloves, and cinnamon; mix with a whisk. Make a well in the center and add the egg substitute and granulated sugar. Add the applesauce and pumpkin, stirring into the egg and sugar. Gradually start to mix into dry ingredients, stirring just until moistened. Fold in the raisins and pecans if using. Spoon into the prepared pan. Bake 1 hour and 15 minutes or until a wooden pick inserted near the center comes out clean.

Mix glaze: In a small bowl, combine the powdered sugar and gradually add the milk, stirring until smooth.

Cool the cake in the pan on a wire rack for 10 minutes. Remove from pan, place flat side down on wire rack, and position the rack and cake over a plate or piece of paper to catch drippings. Drizzle with the glaze, letting it run down the sides slightly.

(continued)

Garnish: Sprinkle with a few chopped pecans, if desired. During the holidays, chopped red and green candied or maraschino cherries would be very pretty. Or use the whole cherries and make clusters of three red cherries, cut a green cherry in fourths, and use these pieces for the leaves, placing one on each side of the clusters of three red cherries. Make either 3 or 5 clusters on the top of the glaze.

PINEAPPLE CAKE

SERVES 10

5.4 GRAMS FAT
PER SERVING

Prep :20
Cook :45
Stand :30
Total :1:35

1 (18-ounce) package 97% fat-free yellow cake mix
1 (14-ounce) can crushed pineapple in light syrup, undrained
2 (3-ounce) packages fat-free vanilla instant pudding mix
4 cups skim milk
1 (8-ounce) container fat-free cream cheese
1 large container Lite Cool Whip, thawed
1 cup unsweetened shredded coconut (optional)
1 cup nuts, chopped (optional)

Prepare the cake mix according to directions on the package, substituting egg substitute for eggs and skim milk for % milk. Pour the batter into a 9 x 13-inch baking pan, sprayed lightly with vegetable oil cooking spray. Bake 35 to 40 minutes, or until done. Cool on a wire rack until completely cool. With a fork, make holes in the cake; spread pineapple, juice and all, evenly over cake.

With a wire whisk, in a mixing bowl, combine the pudding mix with 4 cups of skim milk until it thickens. Stir in cream cheese. Spread evenly over pineapple.

Stir Cool Whip; add coconut and nuts if using. Spread over the pudding mix. Sprinkle a few chopped pecans over the top for decoration, if desired.

FRESH RHUBARB CAKE

½ cup fat-free margarine, at room temperature
1¼ cups sugar
¼ cup egg substitute
1 cup low-fat buttermilk (1 gram per cup)
1 teaspoon vanilla extract
2 cups all-purpose flour
1 teaspoon baking soda
½ teaspoon salt
2 cups chopped rhubarb, frozen or fresh
½ teaspoon ground cinnamon
Dessert Sauce (see below)

SERVES 12

0.5 GRAM FAT
PER SERVING

Prep :15
Cook :40
Stand :00
Total :55

Preheat the oven to 350 degrees. Lightly spray a 13 x 9-inch baking pan with vegetable oil cooking spray.

In a medium-size mixing bowl, cream the margarine and 1 cup of the sugar. Add the egg substitute; beat well. In a small bowl, combine the buttermilk and vanilla. In another bowl, whisk together the flour, baking soda, and salt.

Add one third of the flour to the creamed mixture and beat well. Beat in half the buttermilk. Add another third of the flour, then the rest of the buttermilk, ending with the flour. Stir in the rhubarb.

Spread in the prepared baking pan. Combine the remaining ¼ cup of sugar and the cinnamon and sprinkle over the batter. Bake for 35 to 40 minutes or until the cake tests done with a toothpick. Serve with warm Dessert Sauce.

Dessert Sauce

½ cup sugar
½ cup evaporated skim milk
½ teaspoon vanilla extract
¼ cup Butter Buds

In a small saucepan, combine the above ingredients for the sauce, bring to a boil, and simmer for about 10 minutes. Pour over hot cake. Yum.

Serve with low-fat whipped topping or fat-free frozen yogurt.

CHOCOLATE CAKE AND FROSTING

SERVES 12

**6 GRAMS FAT
ENTIRE CAKE**

**Prep :20
Cook :30
Stand :45
Total 1:35**

2 cups all-purpose flour
2 cups granulated sugar
⅓ cup unsweetened cocoa powder
1½ teaspoons baking soda
1½ cups skim milk
⅓ cup applesauce
1 teaspoon vanilla extract
2 egg whites
Chocolate Frosting (see below)

Preheat the oven to 350 degrees. Spray two 9-inch round baking pans with vegetable oil cooking spray and dust lightly with flour.

In a large mixing bowl, combine the flour, 1¾ cups of the sugar, cocoa, and baking soda. Add the milk, applesauce, and vanilla. Beat with an electric mixer on low speed until well blended. Beat on medium speed for about 2 additional minutes, scraping the sides of the bowl occasionally.

Wash the beaters thoroughly. In a small mixing bowl, beat the egg whites until soft peaks form; gradually add the remaining ¼ cup sugar, beating until stiff peaks form (tips stand straight). Fold into the batter. Pour the batter into the prepared pans.

Bake for 25 to 30 minutes or until a wooden toothpick inserted near the center of the cake comes out clean. Cool the cakes in their pans on wire racks for 10 minutes. Remove the cakes from the pans and cool them thoroughly on wire racks. Frost with Chocolate Frosting.

Chocolate Frosting

2 cups powdered sugar
3 tablespoons unsweetened cocoa powder
1 (8-ounce) package fat-free cream cheese, at room temperature
½ teaspoon vanilla extract

In a medium-size mixing bowl, mix the powdered sugar and 3 tablespoons cocoa; add the softened cream cheese and ½ teaspoon vanilla. Stir with a wire whisk very gently because the fat-free cream cheese will break down and be too thin if you beat it too vigorously. Spread frosting between the layers, then frost the sides and top.

PUMPKIN YUM PIE

½ cup egg substitute
1 (16-ounce) can solid-pack pumpkin
1 (12-ounce) can evaporated skim milk
¼ cup honey
½ cup packed brown sugar
⅓ cup granulated sugar
1 tablespoon pumpkin pie spice
1 unbaked pie shell

Topping:
¼ cup English walnuts, chopped
⅓ cup packed brown sugar

SERVES 6

LOW-FAT

Prep :20
Cook 1:10
Stand :00
Total 1:30

Preheat the oven to 375 degrees.

In a large mixing bowl, whisk together the egg substitute, pumpkin, milk, honey, sugars, and pie spice. Pour into the unbaked pie shell. Bake for 30 minutes.

For the topping, mix the nuts and ⅓ cup brown sugar. Carefully pull the oven rack out and sprinkle the nut mixture over the partially baked pie. Carefully move the rack back and continue baking for an additional 30 to 40 minutes, or until a knife inserted near the center comes out clean. Top with a dollop of light whipped topping. Yum!

FAT-FREE FROZEN YOGURT PIE

Plan on starting this at least one day before you need it.

SERVES 8

0 GRAMS FAT
IF NUTS
OMITTED

Prep :30
Cook 1:00
Stand 1:00
Total 2:30

Meringue Crust:
2 large egg whites, at room temperature
½ teaspoon vanilla extract
¼ teaspoon salt
¼ teaspoon cream of tartar
½ cup sugar
½ cup finely chopped pecans (optional)

Filling:
2 pints frozen yogurt, fat-free of course, choice of flavor
½ cup strawberry preserves (or preserves of choice)
2 tablespoons Kahlúa (may use sherry)
¼ cup chopped pecans (optional)

Preheat the oven to 275 degrees. Lightly coat a 9-inch pie plate with vegetable oil cooking spray.

Meringue Crust: In a grease-free mixing bowl, beat the egg whites, vanilla, salt, and cream of tartar until soft peaks form. Gradually add the sugar, beating until stiff peaks form and sugar is dissolved. Fold in the ½ cup chopped pecans if using. Spread the mixture in the prepared pie plate, building up the sides to form a pie shell effect. Bake for 1 hour, turn off heat, DO NOT OPEN OVEN; let dry in the oven for an additional hour or overnight, keeping the door closed. Cool completely.

Filling: Soften the yogurt to a workable consistency. Arrange scoops of yogurt in the cooled meringue crust (about 8 scoops, 1 in center and 7 around edge). Return to the freezer and freeze for several hours until firm or overnight.

Just before serving, combine preserves and Kahlúa or sherry and drizzle over scoops of yogurt. Sprinkle with the remaining ¼ cup of chopped pecans if desired.

Serve immediately.

CHOCOLATE CHIP COOKIES

2 cups all-purpose flour
1 teaspoon baking soda
¼ teaspoon salt
¼ cup egg substitute
3 tablespoons weak cold coffee
1 teaspoon vanilla extract
¼ cup canola oil
1 cup packed brown sugar
½ cup semisweet chocolate chips

MAKES 36

2.5 GRAMS FAT
PER COOKIE

Prep :25
Cook :08
Stand :03
Total :36

Preheat the oven to 375 degrees. Lightly spray two cookie sheets with vegetable oil cooking spray.

In a mixing bowl, combine the flour, baking soda, and salt. Set aside.

In a small bowl, combine the egg substitute, coffee, and vanilla. Set aside.

In a large mixing bowl, blend the canola oil and brown sugar with an electric mixer on low speed. Add the egg substitute mixture. Beat until smooth. Add the flour mixture in two parts at low speed. Scrape the bowl well after each addition. Stir in the chocolate chips by hand.

Drop by rounded teaspoonfuls onto the prepared baking sheets. Bake for 7 to 8 minutes or until lightly browned. Cool on baking sheets for 1 minute and remove with a spatula to a wire cooling rack for an additional 2 minutes, if you can wait that long.

SUGAR COOKIES

**MAKES
ABOUT 3
DOZEN**

0 GRAMS FAT

**Prep :25
Cook :10
Stand :03
Total :38**

2 cups all-purpose flour
1½ teaspoons baking soda
1 cup sugar, plus additional as needed
½ cup fat-free margarine, at room temperature
1 teaspoon vanilla extract
¼ cup egg substitute

Preheat the oven to 375 degrees. Spray two baking sheets lightly with vegetable oil cooking spray.

In a small bowl combine the flour and baking soda, mix well, and set aside.

In a medium bowl, with an electric mixer at medium speed, beat 1 cup of sugar, the margarine, and vanilla until creamy. Add the egg substitute and mix well.

Stir in the flour mixture until blended. Shape the dough into balls, and roll in sugar if desired. (I desired!) Place about 2 inches apart on the prepared pans. Bake for 8 to 10 minutes, or until light brown. We like them at the geriatric stage (soft). Cool on a wire rack.

Variations:
- Add a tablespoon of cinnamon to the sugar that I roll them in.
- Add a teaspoon of cinnamon to the dough.
- Add a teaspoon of grated orange zest to the dough.
- Add a cup of chopped pecans. This gives them the snickerdoodle taste if you roll them in the cinnamon sugar. (You have added some fat grams when you add the pecans.)

OATMEAL COOKIES

1 cup all-purpose flour
½ cup sugar
1 cup quick-cooking rolled oats
¼ teaspoon salt (optional)
½ teaspoon baking powder
½ teaspoon baking soda
½ teaspoon cinnamon
¼ teaspoon ground nutmeg
2 egg whites
⅓ cup light corn syrup
1 teaspoon vanilla extract
½ cup raisins
½ cup walnuts, chopped (optional)

MAKES
ABOUT 3
DOZEN

0 GRAMS FAT
WITHOUT
NUTS

Prep: :15
Cook :10
Stand .00
Total :25

Preheat the oven to 375 degrees. Spray one or two baking sheets lightly with vegetable oil cooking spray.

In a large bowl, combine the flour, sugar, oats, salt if desired, baking powder, baking soda, cinnamon, and nutmeg.

Stir in the unbeaten egg whites, corn syrup, and vanilla. Mix well, then add raisins, and the walnuts if desired.

Drop teaspoonfuls of the dough 1 inch apart on the prepared baking sheets. Bake for 10 minutes. *Do not overbake.* Remove with a spatula and cool the cookies on a rack.

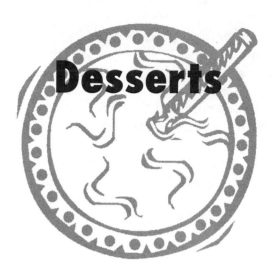

Desserts

PUMPKIN DELIGHT

SERVES 6

VERY LOW-FAT

Prep :15
Cook :00
Stand :30
Total :45

1 (3-ounce) package sugar-free instant pudding mix
1½ cups skim milk
1 cup canned pumpkin
1 teaspoon pumpkin pie spice
1½ cups lite whipped topping, thawed, plus additional as needed
1 low-fat graham cracker crust or prebaked pie shell

In a mixing bowl, beat the pudding mix and milk until well blended. Blend in the pumpkin and pie spice; fold in the 1½ cups of topping. Spoon into pie shell and chill. Dollop with light topping for garnish, and sprinkle a little ginger on dollops of topping.

> *Variations:* No-Crust Pumpkin Delight: Spoon into dessert dishes, chill, and serve with a nonfat cookie.
> Add pecans if desired (it will add fat grams). Chop ½ cup pecans fine and stir in just before spooning the pudding into the dish or pie shell.

"I WORKED ALL DAY MAKING THIS DESSERT!"

1 GRAM FAT PER SERVING

Prep :05
Cook :00
Stand 1:00
Total 1:05

Angel food cake, cubed
Fat-free frozen yogurt or ice cream
Kahlúa
Lite whipped topping
Chopped pecans or maraschino cherries

Several hours before serving time, place a layer of cake cubes in the bottom of individual dessert dishes. On top of the cake, scoop about two scoops of frozen yogurt or ice cream of your desired flavor (chocolate is very good for this dessert, and mixing flavors such as strawberry and chocolate is also tasty as well as pretty). You may wish to add a layer of cake between the scoops of yogurt or ice cream. Pour about ¼ cup Kahlúa over each (more or less may be used; do your own thing). Place the dishes in the freezer for at least 1 hour, or until time to serve. Pour about 1 tablespoon more Kahlúa over each dessert, top with a scoop of lite whipped topping that has been thawed in the refrigerator, sprinkle chopped pecans over or top with a maraschino cherry (the one with the long stem still on is very attractive). Your guests will love this.

Use a pretty dessert dish, to complement the season or occasion. It will be frosted when served, which adds to the attractiveness. It does look like you worked all day—don't say a word! They will wonder what the Kahlúa is.

CHOCOLATE BREAD PUDDING

I usually serve this at room temperature, but it is also good served hot or cold.

SERVES 4

2.5 GRAMS FAT
PER SERVING

Prep :20
Cook :45
Stand :00
Total 1:05

1½ cups evaporated skim milk
½ cup sugar
4 teaspoons unsweetened cocoa powder
1 teaspoon vanilla extract
¾ cup egg substitute
3½ cups (½-inch) cubed French bread
2 tablespoons semisweet chocolate mini-morsels

Preheat the oven to 325 degrees. Lightly spray four 6-ounce custard cups with vegetable oil cooking spray.

In a mixing bowl, combine the milk, sugar, and cocoa. Stir with a wire whisk until blended. Add the vanilla and egg substitute; stir well. Add the bread cubes, stirring until moistened. Spoon the mixture evenly into the prepared custard cups. Top with mini-morsels.

(continued)

Place the cups in a 9 x 13-inch baking pan. Add about 1 inch of hot water to the pan. Bake for 40 to 45 minutes or until a knife inserted in the center comes out clean.

> *Variation:* The pudding may be baked in a 2-quart baking dish set in a 9 x 13-inch pan. Lightly spray the baking dish with vegetable oil cooking spray. Heat the oven to 375 degrees and add hot water to the pan to a depth of 1½ inches. Bake 40 to 45 minutes.

LEMON BREAD PUDDING

SERVES 4

2.5 GRAMS FAT
PER 1-CUP
SERVING

Prep :20
Cook :55
Stand 1:00
Total 2:15

1¾ cups buttermilk (skim or 1 gram fat per cup)
¾ cup sugar
¾ cup egg substitute
⅓ cup lemon juice
2 tablespoons Butter Buds, liquid form
2 teaspoons grated lemon rind
8 (½-inch) slices French bread, cut into 1-inch squares

Preheat the oven to 350 degrees. Lightly spray a 2-quart round or an 11 x 7-inch baking dish with vegetable oil cooking spray. Set aside.

Combine the buttermilk, sugar, egg substitute, lemon juice, Butter Buds, and grated lemon rind in a large mixing bowl. Add the bread cubes and toss to mix well. Let stand about 1 hour.

Spoon the mixture into the prepared baking dish and bake at 350 degrees for 50 to 55 minutes or until the pudding is set. Serve warm or at room temperature with Lemon Sauce (page 199).

> *Tip:* Lemon instant pudding mix is fast and easy to finish off your dessert as well as fat-free. (Read your labels!) Add about ½ cup extra liquid for a thinner consistency for ladling over pudding.
> Lemon regular pudding mix, cooked according to directions, is also fat-free and wonderful over the pudding. Add about ½ cup extra liquid for a thinner consistency for ladling over pudding.

LOW-FAT, SUGAR-FREE BREAD PUDDING

A great do-ahead dish.

SERVES 4

7 GRAMS FAT
ENTIRE DISH

Prep :10
Cook :07
Stand 8:00
Total 8:17

8 thin slices low-fat white bread, crusts removed
3 cups fresh berries, or 1 (12-ounce) package frozen dry-pack berries, such as raspberries, blackberries, or blueberries (reserve 4 for garnish)
1 (4-ounce) can crushed pineapple, drained, with ⅓ cup juice reserved

Lightly spray a deep 4-cup dish or pudding mold with vegetable oil cooking spray. Line the bottom and sides with 7 slices of the bread, overlapping them slightly.

In a medium-size heavy saucepan, bring the berries, pineapple, and reserved juice to a boil over moderately high heat for about 2 minutes. Lower the heat and simmer for 4 additional minutes.

Spoon the fruit mixture into the prepared dish and top with the remaining slice of bread. Cover with waxed paper and place a weight, such as a plate weighted down with cans of food, on top. Refrigerate overnight.

To serve: Loosen with a thin-bladed metal spatula and invert onto a serving plate. Serve plain or with nonfat frozen yogurt, ice cream, or lite whipped topping.

Place the reserved berries on the top of whatever you are serving the pudding with.

TOASTY APPLE BREAD PUDDING

This pudding is equally good served warm or cold.

SERVES 8

0.5 GRAM FAT
PER SERVING

Prep :10
Cook :45
Stand :10
Total 1:05

4 slices low-fat bread (1 gram per slice)
2 apples, peeled, cored, and chopped
1/2 cup egg substitute
1/2 cup sugar (or sugar substitute, such as Sugar Twin)
1 cup evaporated skim milk
1/2 cup applesauce
1 teaspoon vanilla extract
1 teaspoon ground cinnamon

Preheat the oven to 350 degrees. Lightly spray a 1 1/2-quart baking dish with vegetable oil cooking spray.

Toast the bread slices, cut into 1/2-inch cubes, and place in the prepared baking dish. Add the chopped apples.

In a separate bowl, mix the egg substitute, 1/4 cup of the sugar, the milk, applesauce, and the 1/2 cup water. Mix with a wire whisk. Pour over the bread and apples. Let stand for 8 to 10 minutes. Stir in the vanilla.

Mix the remaining 1/4 cup of sugar with the cinnamon. Sprinkle over the top of the pudding mixture.

Bake for 40 to 45 minutes or until a knife inserted in the center comes out clean.

OLD-FASHIONED BANANA PUDDING

This can be sugar-free as well as almost fat-free.

½ cup plus 1 tablespoon sugar or sugar substitute
3 tablespoons cornstarch
⅓ cup water
1 (12-ounce) can evaporated skim milk
⅓ cup egg substitute
½ cup fat-free sour cream
1 teaspoon vanilla extract
25 vanilla wafers
3 medium bananas, sliced
3 egg whites
¼ teaspoon cream of tartar

SERVES 8

LESS THAN 1
GRAM FAT PER
SERVING

Prep :30
Cook :30
Stand :00
Total 1:00

Preheat the oven to 325 degrees.

In a heavy saucepan, combine the ½ cup of sugar (or sugar substitute) with the cornstarch. Gradually stir in ⅓ cup of water, the milk, and the egg substitute. Cook over medium heat, stirring constantly, until the mixture comes to a boil. Lower the heat and boil for 1 minute, stirring constantly. Remove from the heat and fold in the sour cream and vanilla.

In an ovenproof baking dish (about a 1½-quart), arrange a layer of vanilla wafers, about ⅓ of the pudding mix, and a layer of bananas. Repeat the layers, ending with vanilla wafers. (You may end with just pudding, but I like more cookies in my banana pudding.)

In a medium-size mixing bowl, free of grease, beat the egg whites and cream of tartar until foamy. Gradually add the 1 tablespoon sugar (or sugar substitute), beating until stiff peaks form. Spread the meringue over the pudding, making sure the meringue touches all edges of the baking dish.

Bake for 25 to 30 minutes, until the meringue is golden. Let cool to room temperature or serve cold.

Your guests will think Grandma is here for sure. I don't know of a grandma in the world who doesn't make banana pudding for the little darlings.

BAKED RICE PUDDING

SERVES 4

LESS THAN 1
GRAM FAT PER
SERVING

Prep :20
Cook :55
Stand :00
Total 1:15

3 egg whites
¼ cup egg substitute
1½ cups skim milk
¼ cup sugar
1 teaspoon vanilla extract
⅔ cup cooked rice
2 tablespoons raisins (optional)
Ground cinnamon (optional)

Preheat the oven to 325 degrees. Lightly coat a 1½-quart casserole with vegetable oil cooking spray.

In a medium-size mixing bowl, combine the egg whites, egg substitute, milk, sugar, and vanilla. Beat until well combined but not foamy. Stir in the cooked rice and raisins, if desired. (I do not use raisins—I don't like them—but they are good in this recipe.) Pour egg mixture into the prepared casserole. Place the casserole in a baking pan and add boiling water to the pan to a depth of about 1 inch.

Bake uncovered for 45 to 55 minutes or until just moist, stirring after 35 minutes. Serve warm or chilled. Sprinkle with cinnamon if desired.

STOVETOP RICE PUDDING

2 cups skim milk
¼ cup long-grain rice
2 tablespoons raisins (optional)
¼ cup sugar
1 teaspoon vanilla
Cinnamon (optional)

SERVES 4

LESS THAN 1
GRAM FAT PER
½-CUP
SERVING

Prep :10
Cook :40
Stand :00
Total :50

In a heavy saucepan, bring the milk to a boil and stir in the uncooked rice and raisins, if desired. Cover and cook over low heat, stirring occasionally, for 30 to 40 minutes or until most of the milk is absorbed. (Mixture may appear curdled.) Stir in sugar and vanilla. Spoon into dessert dishes.

Serve warm or chilled. If desired, sprinkle with ground cinnamon.

AMARETTO RICE PUDDING

¾ cup egg substitute
⅔ cup sugar
¼ teaspoon salt
2 cups skim milk
1 cup uncooked instant rice
¼ teaspoon cinnamon
¼ cup coconut amaretto or plain amaretto
1 teaspoon vanilla extract
2 tablespoons raisins (optional)
Ground nutmeg for sprinkling over top (optional)

SERVES 6

LESS THAN 1
GRAM FAT PER
¾-CUP
SERVING

Prep :15
Cook :50
Stand :00
Total 1:05

Preheat the oven to 325 degrees. Lightly coat a 1½-quart baking dish with vegetable oil cooking spray.

In a large mixing bowl, combine the egg substitute, sugar, salt, milk, rice, cinnamon, amaretto, and vanilla extract. Stir in raisins, if desired. *(continued)*

Pour into the prepared baking dish. Place in a larger shallow baking dish; pour hot water into the pan about 1 inch deep.

Bake for 30 minutes. Stir, sprinkle with nutmeg if desired, and continue baking for 20 additional minutes. Serve the pudding warm or cool. Drizzle about 2 tablespoons of amaretto over the top before serving if desired.

FRUIT CRISP

You can use in-season fruit such as apples, cherries, blueberries, peaches, or pears; or use any fruit pie filling, such as cherry, apple, or peach.

SERVES 4

0 GRAMS FAT

Prep :20
Cook :40
Stand :00
Total 1:00

2 tablespoons lemon juice
2 to 3 cups peeled and chopped fruit
¾ cup packed brown sugar
2 tablespoons cornstarch
⅔ cup quick-cooking rolled oats
½ cup all-purpose flour
½ cup Butter Buds, liquid form
Fat-free frozen yogurt or ice cream (optional)

Preheat the oven to 350 degrees. Lightly spray a 1½-quart baking dish with vegetable oil cooking spray.

Add lemon juice to the fruit and stir to coat. Combine ¼ cup of the brown sugar and the cornstarch; add to fruit mixture. Spoon into the prepared baking dish. If using pie filling, pour directly into prepared baking dish.

In a separate mixing bowl, combine the remaining ½ cup of brown sugar, the oats, and flour. Mix. Stream Butter Buds over the oat mixture; stir to mix until it looks like coarse meal. Sprinkle mixture over fruit. Bake for 30 to 40 minutes. Serve with fat-free frozen yogurt or ice cream if desired. Yummy in your tummy!

CHOCOLATE SAUCE

1 cup sugar
6 tablespoons skim milk
2 tablespoons unsweetened cocoa powder
2 tablespoons light corn syrup
2 teaspoons vanilla extract

SERVES 2

TRACE OF FAT

Prep :05
Cook :01
Stand :00
Total :06

In a heavy saucepan, combine the sugar, milk, cocoa, and corn syrup. Bring to a boil; boil 1 minute. Remove from heat; stir in vanilla.

Serve as a fruit dip or over fat-free ice cream, frozen yogurt, your favorite dessert, such as bread pudding, or a heavy-type cake.

LEMON SAUCE

½ cup sugar
2 tablespoons cornstarch
¼ cup lemon juice
½ teaspoon grated lemon rind

MAKES
1 ½ CUPS

0 GRAMS FAT

Prep :05
Cook :03
Stand :00
Total :08

In a small heavy saucepan, combine the sugar and cornstarch, blend with a whisk, and gradually add 1¼ cups of water and the lemon juice. Set over medium heat, bring to a boil, reduce heat, and cook, stirring constantly, until the sauce has thickened and is clear, about 2 or 3 minutes.

Remove from the heat, cool, and stir in the lemon rind. Serve over puddings or any dessert.

The sauce may be stored tightly covered up to 1 week in the refrigerator.

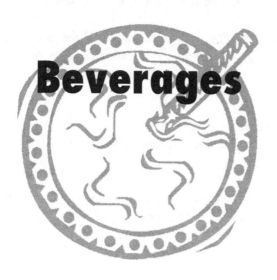

Beverages

LEMON-LIME PUNCH

Very pretty, as well as good for weddings or showers. The color is nice for spring and summertime.

SERVES 20

0 GRAMS FAT

Prep :05
Cook :00
Stand :00
Total :05

1 pint lemon sherbet
1 (28-ounce) can pineapple juice, chilled
1 (28-ounce) can lemon-lime-flavor carbonated beverage, chilled
1 pint lime sherbet

Blend the lemon sherbet with the pineapple juice in a punch bowl. Stir in the lemon-lime beverage and spoon the lime sherbet on top. Makes about 20 cup servings.

FROSTY WINE SLUSH

SERVES 4

0 GRAMS FAT

Prep :10
Cook :00
Stand :00
Total :10

1 pint frozen fat-free fruit sorbet
1 cup dry white wine
2 tablespoons lemon juice
1 cup crushed ice
Lime wedges for garnish (optional)

In a blender container, combine the first three ingredients; blend until mixed. Add the ice and blend until slushy. Pour into chilled cocktail glasses. Garnish with lime wedges if desired.

SNAPPY TOMATO SIPPER

4 cups cold tomato juice
¼ cup lime or lemon juice
2 teaspoons Worcestershire sauce
2 to 4 drops hot sauce
½ cup vodka
Garnish: celery stalks with leaves

SERVES 2

0 GRAMS FAT

Prep :05
Cook :00
Stand :00
Total :05

Combine the first three ingredients in a pitcher, blending well. Stir in a couple drops of hot sauce, taste, and add more if desired. Stir in vodka. Chill. Garnish with a celery stalk used as a stirrer in each glass.

LEMON-LIME FROZEN DAIQUIRIS

1 (14-ounce) can frozen lemonade concentrate
½ lemonade can light rum
3 drops green food coloring
5 to 6 cups ice
¼ cup lime juice (optional)
Fresh lime slices (optional)

SERVES 2

0 GRAMS FAT

Prep :10
Cook :00
Stand :00
Total :10

Put the frozen lemonade concentrate in a blender container and add the rum and green food coloring. Blend to a smooth consistency. Add ice, a cup at a time, until as thick as you like. Add lime juice if desired, and blend about 5 seconds longer.

Pour into cocktail glasses and garnish with a slice of lime on the rim if desired.

I usually make a double batch of these and store in a wide-mouth plastic container in the freezer. You can dip out as many as you want anytime you want.

FROZEN MARGARITAS, MIDWESTERN STYLE

SERVES 4

0 GRAMS FAT

Prep :10
Cook :00
Stand :00
Total :10

1 (14-ounce) can frozen limeade concentrate (or you can use lemonade)
¾ limeade can tequila
¼ cup triple sec
4 to 6 cups ice
Fresh lime, cut into small triangle pieces
Coarse salt

Put the frozen limeade concentrate in a blender container. Blend long enough to liquefy. Add tequila and triple sec and start adding ice a cup at a time, blending until the desired consistency.

Prepare cocktail glasses by rubbing the rims with a cut lime, then dipping the rims into a saucer of coarse salt.

Fill the glasses with margaritas, squeeze a lime section over top of each glass, and add that piece of lime to the top. I make two or three batches of these ahead of time before entertaining, place them in the freezer, and am free to visit with my guests. We can dip just as many as desired when desired. Leftovers are wonderful later without any effort.

MULLED CIDER

SERVES 4

0 GRAMS FAT

Prep :10
Cook :15
Stand :00
Total :25

1 quart apple cider
⅓ cup packed brown sugar
½ teaspoon whole allspice
6 to 7 (3-inch) cinnamon sticks
6 to 7 whole cloves

In a large saucepan or dutch oven, combine the apple cider with the brown sugar, allspice, cloves, and 2 or 3 cinnamon sticks. Bring to a boil, reduce the heat, cover, and simmer for 15 minutes. Remove and discard spices. Serve hot with a cinnamon stick standing up in each cup.

CHRISTMAS WASSAIL

The fragrance in the house during the holidays makes this worth making whether you drink it or not.

SERVES 10

0 GRAMS FAT

Prep :10
Cook :15
Stand :00
Total :25

½ gallon apple cider
4 cups orange juice (fresh is nice and in season at Christmas)
⅓ cup lemon juice (about 2 lemons and also in season)
½ cup honey
4 to 5 (3-inch) cinnamon sticks
¼ teaspoon ground nutmeg

In a large saucepan or dutch oven, combine all ingredients. Bring to a boil over medium heat. Remove and discard the cinnamon sticks; serve hot. Makes about 14 cups.

YE OLD WASSAIL

Christmas memories are added to with the aroma of this drink brewing. When your guests walk in they will be sure they are going to see chestnuts roasting over an open fire.

SERVES 12

0 GRAMS FAT

Prep :10
Cook 2:00
Stand :00
Total 2:10

2 oranges
40 whole cloves
1 gallon apple cider
⅔ of 1 (46-ounce) can pineapple juice
⅔ of 1 (6-ounce) can frozen orange juice concentrate
Juice of 2 lemons
¾ box or jar of cinnamon sticks

Stud the oranges with cloves. In a large kettle, combine the cider with the pineapple, orange, and lemon juices. Add the cinnamon sticks and clove-studded oranges. Bring to a boil and simmer for 1½ to 2 hours before time to serve.

LEGAL EGGNOG

Who said we can't have any eggnog!

SERVES 4

0 GRAMS FAT

Prep :15
Cook :00
Stand :00
Total :15

1 (12-ounce) can evaporated skim milk, chilled
1 teaspoon rum or brandy extract (2 tablespoons rum or brandy)
4 teaspoons sugar
2 large egg whites
Freshly grated nutmeg

Combine the milk, rum, and sugar in a medium-size bowl. Stir until the sugar is dissolved.

In another medium bowl, free of any grease and chilled, beat the egg whites until they hold soft peaks, then fold into the milk mixture.

Ladle into chilled punch cups or wine glasses and sprinkle with nutmeg.

HOT SPICED TEA MIX

SERVES 32

0 GRAMS FAT

Prep :10
Cook :00
Stand :00
Total :10

This makes a nice gift for a special friend. Pack in a pretty glass container or a glass quart jar and decorate the top by cutting a piece of fabric, with pinking shears, in an 8-inch circle. Place a little piece of cotton or a couple of cotton balls, pulled a little to flatten out, on the lid, cover with fabric, place the ring over, and screw on. Leave the fabric hanging down like a little ruffle. Quick and easy. Choose a scrap of fabric that complements the receiver's kitchen.

2 cups instant orange-flavored breakfast drink (such as Tang)
2 cups sugar
½ cup instant tea
1 (0.31-ounce) package unsweetened lemon-flavored drink mix

1 teaspoon ground cinnamon
1 teaspoon ground cloves
Garnish: cinnamon sticks (optional)

Combine all ingredients except cinnamon sticks. Mix well.

To serve: For each serving, place 1½ to 2 tablespoons of the mix in a cup, add boiling water, and stir well. Garnish if desired with a cinnamon stick in each cup.

To store: Store in an airtight container at room temperature for up to 3 months.

RUSSIAN TEA

Remember this recipe from way back when? It is a nice from-the-heart, for-the-heart gift. Use the gift jar idea from the recipe for Hot Spiced Tea Mix on page 206.

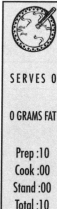

SERVES 0

0 GRAMS FAT

Prep :10
Cook :00
Stand :00
Total :10

½ cup instant tea
2 cups instant orange drink mix
1½ cups sugar
1 teaspoon ground cinnamon
½ teaspoon ground cloves

Mix all the above ingredients; store in an airtight container.

To serve: Spoon 3½ teaspoons into each cup; fill cups with hot water.

Make a little nametag-like card with instructions for serving and attach to each gift container.

HOT CHOCOLATE COFFEE

SERVES 1

0 GRAMS FAT

Prep :01
Cook :00
Stand :00
Total :01

1 teaspoon instant coffee
1 (0.53-ounce) package Swiss Miss sugar-free fat-free cocoa mix
1 cup hot water
1 cinnamon stick (optional)

Place the coffee and cocoa mix in a cup; add hot water; stir well to blend. Add a stick of cinnamon if desired.

HOT CHOCOLATE MIX

Makes a great gift. Follow the instructions for decorating the container in the Hot Spiced Tea Mix recipe on page 206.

MAKES 32
SERVINGS

TRACE OF FAT
IN EACH
SERVING

Prep :10
Cook :00
Stand :00
Total :10

2¼ cups powdered sugar
2 cups nonfat dry milk powder
2 cups powdered fat-free nondairy coffee creamer
2 cups chocolate milk mix
¾ cup instant coffee granules
3 tablespoons ground cinnamon
Garnish: cinnamon sticks

Combine all ingredients except the cinnamon sticks. Stir well.
To serve: For each serving, spoon ¼ cup mix into a cup, fill the cup with boiling water, and stir well. Garnish if desired with a cinnamon stick.
To store: Store in an airtight container at room temperature for up to 3 months.

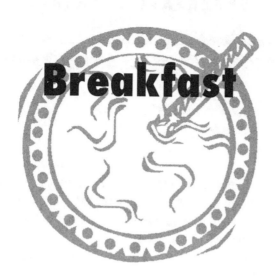

Breakfast

BREAKFAST COCKTAIL

Place your champagne glasses in the freezer or refrigerator the night before to make this drink look prettier.

SERVES 4

0 GRAMS FAT

Prep :10
Cook :00
Stand :00
Total :10

2 cups sliced fresh peaches or thawed frozen peaches
⅔ cup peach or apricot nectar
Champagne

In the container of an electric blender, combine the peaches and nectar. Cover and process until smooth. (May be blended up to a week ahead and stored in an airtight container in the freezer. Remove 30 minutes before serving.)

To serve: Spoon about ⅔ cup of the peach mixture into a stemmed champagne glass. Add about ⅔ cup of champagne to each glass.

Variation: This may also be done with strawberries. Substitute berries for peaches, and grenadine for nectar. Very pretty during the Christmas holidays. I also save 4 fresh berries, if using fresh, and float in the top of each, especially during the summer. Cool and fresh looking. If using frozen berries, a green maraschino cherry is pretty for a seasonal touch.

CHAMPAGNE ORANGE JUICE

SERVES 4

0 GRAMS FAT

Prep :05
Cook :00
Stand :00
Total :05

1 (6-ounce) can frozen orange juice concentrate
1 cup cold water
2½ cups cold champagne
2 thin slices of orange, cut in half and split for garnish

In a glass pitcher or container, mix the orange juice concentrate and water. Stir well. Just before serving, slowly add champagne and stir gently to blend. Pour into champagne glasses and garnish with orange slices on the rim. (Chilled glasses add a nice touch.)

FAT-FREE PANCAKES

SERVES 8

0 GRAMS FAT

Prep :10
Cook :10
Stand :00
Total :20

1¼ cups all-purpose flour
2½ teaspoons baking powder
½ teaspoon salt
¼ cup egg substitute
1¼ cups skim milk

In a mixing bowl, combine the flour, baking powder, and salt. Mix well. In a small bowl, mix together the egg substitute and milk. Stir into the flour mixture just until moistened. (Batter will be lumpy.)

Spray a nonstick skillet lightly with vegetable oil cooking spray. Heat to medium hot. Spoon the batter into hot skillet to make pancakes about 4 inches in diameter.

Cook until bubbles form on the surface, turn with a spatula, and continue to cook until the bottom is golden brown. Serve with hot or warm syrup.

Tip: While you are mixing and cooking your pancakes, place your syrup bottle in a bowl or pan full of very hot water. By the time you are ready the syrup will be nice and warm.

Variation: Whole-Wheat Pancakes: Follow directions above, substituting an equal quantity of whole-wheat flour for the all-purpose flour (or use a mixture of whole-wheat and white). Increase the milk to 1½ cups.

DE "LITE" FUL ZERO-FAT PANCAKES

SERVES 4

0 GRAMS FAT

Prep :10
Cook :10
Stand :00
Total :20

½ cup egg substitute
1 cup fat-free cottage cheese
⅔ cup skim milk
½ teaspoon vanilla extract
1 cup all-purpose flour
½ teaspoon baking soda
Pinch of salt (optional)

In a blender or the bowl of an electric mixer, combine the egg substitute, cottage cheese, milk, and vanilla. Mix until smooth. Add the flour, baking soda, and salt, if desired. On low speed, continue just until mixed.

Lightly spray a large nonstick skillet or griddle with vegetable oil cooking spray; heat over medium heat. Ladle the batter onto the skillet to form 4-inch pancakes. Cook until bubbles form on surface. Turn; cook the other side until golden brown. Serve with warm syrup.

MAPLE FRENCH TOAST

SERVES 4

1 GRAM FAT
PER SLICE

Prep :10
Cook :12
Stand :00
Total :22

2 large egg whites, lightly beaten
⅔ cup skim milk
1 teaspoon maple extract
8 slices whole-wheat bread

Preheat the oven to 200 degrees.

In a shallow bowl or pie pan, whisk together the egg whites, milk, and maple flavoring until just blended. Spray a nonstick skillet lightly with vegetable oil cooking spray; heat to medium heat.

Quickly dip bread slices in the egg mixture, turning to coat both sides. Place in the skillet and cook about 3 minutes on each side, or until golden brown. (Just dip the number of slices that will fit in your skillet; don't do them all at once—they get too mushy.) As the slices are cooked, place on a platter in the oven to keep warm until serving time.

Serve with hot syrup.

Variation: Substitute 1 teaspoon ground cinnamon, ¼ teaspoon ground nutmeg, and ½ teaspoon vanilla extract for the maple flavoring. This makes a nice spicy toast.

CHRISTMAS MORNING FRENCH TOAST

1 cup packed brown sugar
2 tablespoons light maple syrup
2 large tart apples, peeled and sliced ¼ inch thick
¾ cup egg substitute
1 cup skim milk
1 teaspoon vanilla extract
8 (¾-inch) slices day-old French bread

Syrup:
1 cup applesauce
1 (10-ounce) jar apple jelly
½ teaspoon ground cinnamon
⅛ teaspoon ground cloves

SERVES 8

ABOUT 1 TO
1.5 GRAMS FAT
PER SLICE

Prep :20
Cook :40
Stand 8:30
Total 9:30

Preheat the oven to 350 degrees.

In a small saucepan, boil together the brown sugar, maple syrup, and ½ cup of water until slightly thick. Pour into an ungreased 9 x 13-inch baking dish; arrange the apples on top.

In a mixing bowl, lightly beat the egg substitute, milk, and vanilla. Dip the bread slices into the egg mixture for 1 minute; place over apples. Cover and refrigerate overnight. Remove from the refrigerator 30 minutes before baking.

Bake, uncovered, for 35 to 40 minutes, or until puffy and golden brown. *(continued)*

Syrup

Combine the applesauce, jelly, cinnamon, and cloves in a medium saucepan; cook and stir until hot. May be made the day ahead as is the toast; just warm it while the toast cooks. Pour the warm syrup into a gravy boat and pass at the table.

SAUSAGE AND GRITS
FOR BREAKFAST

Make ahead, cover, and refrigerate
8 hours or more.

SERVES 8

6.75 GRAMS FAT PER SERVING

Prep :25
Cook :62
Stand :00
Total 1:27

1½ pounds low-fat sausage (3 grams per patty), crumbled
½ cup quick-cooking grits, uncooked
3 cups shredded fat-free sharp Cheddar cheese
1 cup egg substitute
1 cup skim milk
½ teaspoon thyme leaves
⅛ teaspoon garlic powder
Garnishes: parsley sprigs, orange slices

Preheat the oven to 350 degrees.

In a nonstick skillet, brown the sausage over medium-low heat, stirring to break up lumps. Transfer to a colander and rinse with hot water to remove all traces of fat. Drain well.

Bring 2 cups of water to a boil in a medium-size saucepan; stir in the grits. Return to a boil, reducing the heat to low, and continue cooking for about 4 minutes, stirring occasionally. Add the cheese, stirring until melted.

In a mixing bowl, combine the egg substitute, milk, thyme, and garlic powder; stir well. Gently and slowly stir the grits mixture into the egg mixture, stirring constantly. Stir in the sausage. Pour into an 11 x 7-inch baking dish lightly sprayed with vegetable oil cooking spray.

Bake uncovered at 350 degrees for 50 to 55 minutes or until set. Garnish with parsley sprigs and orange slices.

BLUEBERRY BREAKFAST BAKE

Great do-ahead for holiday entertaining

¼ cup egg substitute
⅓ cup packed brown sugar
1 cup skim milk
1 teaspoon ground cinnamon
1 teaspoon grated lemon rind
Pinch of ground nutmeg
1 teaspoon vanilla extract
6 slices whole-wheat bread
2 cups frozen dry-pack or fresh blueberries, sorted and stemmed

SERVES 6

LESS THAN 1
GRAM FAT PER
SERVING

Prep :15
Cook :40
Stand 1:00
Total 1:55

In a large bowl, beat the egg substitute and sugar together with a fork until well blended. Stir in the milk, cinnamon, lemon rind, nutmeg, and vanilla. Tear the bread into ½-inch pieces and stir into the mixture. Cover and refrigerate at least 1 hour or overnight.

Preheat the oven to 375 degrees. Lightly coat an 8 x 8-inch baking dish with vegetable oil cooking spray. Stir the blueberries into the bread mixture and spoon into the pan, spreading evenly.

Bake for 40 to 45 minutes, until firm. Serve warm. Sprinkle with a little powdered sugar for garnish.

COFFEE CAKE

Make this the night before and bake while the family is getting up. Nice for the holidays or for brunch.

MAKES 9 SERVINGS

1 GRAM FAT PER SERVING

Prep :10
Cook :40
Stand :00
Total :50

1½ cups all-purpose flour
1 teaspoon baking powder
½ teaspoon baking soda
½ teaspoon salt (optional)
1½ cups bran flakes cereal with raisins
½ cup sugar or sugar substitute
1 cup low-fat buttermilk (1 gram per cup)
¼ cup Butter Buds, liquid form
¼ cup egg substitute

Topping:
2 tablespoons sugar or sugar substitute
½ teaspoon cinnamon

Preheat the oven to 400 degrees. Lightly spray an 8-inch-square pan with vegetable oil cooking spray.

In a large bowl, combine the flour, baking powder, baking soda, and salt, if desired. Stir with a wire whisk to blend. Mix in the bran flakes, sugar, buttermilk, Butter Buds, and egg substitute, stirring just until moistened. Spread the batter in the prepared pan.

Combine topping ingredients; sprinkle over the batter. Bake 30 to 40 minutes or until a toothpick inserted in the center comes out clean. Serve warm.

Note: If making ahead, cover with plastic wrap after adding the topping and refrigerate until baking time.

BAKED GRITS

1½ cups fat-free chicken broth
1½ cups skim milk
⅔ cup hominy grits
¼ teaspoon salt
¼ cup egg substitute
1 large egg white
Dash pepper
1 teaspoon Butter Buds, liquid form

SERVES 4

0 GRAMS FAT

Prep :15
Cook 1:05
Stand :05
Total 1:25

Preheat the oven to 350 degrees. Lightly spray a 1½-quart baking dish with vegetable oil cooking spray. Set aside.

In a medium-size heavy saucepan, bring the chicken broth and 1 cup of the milk to a boil. Stir in the grits and salt, reduce the heat to low, and cook, stirring, for 5 minutes or until thickened. Let cool for about 5 minutes.

In a small bowl, whisk together the remaining ½ cup of milk, the egg substitute, and egg white. Stir the egg mixture into the grits along with pepper and Butter Buds. Spoon the grits into the baking dish and bake uncovered for 1 hour or until golden brown.

Note: May make a day ahead, cool completely, cover with plastic wrap, and refrigerate. Bake as directed.

Variations: Add ¼ cup each sautéed onions and peppers. Or sprinkle ½ cup fat-free shredded cheese over the top; bake an additional 3 to 4 minutes or until cheese is melted. Cheese and/or chopped green chiles may be added to the mixture with either variation before baking. This is a recipe you can have fun and be creative with.

HASH BROWN BREAKFAST CASEROLE

SERVES 8

0 GRAMS FAT

Prep :10
Cook :45
Stand :00
Total :55

1 (10-ounce) package fat-free frozen hash brown potatoes
¼ cup chopped onion
¼ cup chopped bell pepper
½ cup shredded fat-free cheese
1 cup plain nonfat yogurt
1 cup fat-free sour cream
½ cup chopped green chiles (optional)
Salt and pepper to taste

Preheat the oven to 350 degrees. Lightly spray a 9 x 9-inch baking dish with vegetable oil cooking spray.

Combine the potatoes, onions, bell peppers, cheese, yogurt, and sour cream. (If desired include green chiles, especially if you are serving a Western theme breakfast, or breakfast on the patio or deck.) Season to taste with salt and pepper. Mix well and spoon into the prepared baking dish.

Bake uncovered for 40 to 50 minutes or until golden brown.

Note: The casserole may be mixed a day ahead, covered with plastic wrap, and refrigerated until time to cook.

BREAKFAST ROLL-UPS

4 thin slices lean Canadian bacon, chopped
1½ cups fat-free frozen hash brown potatoes
Salt and pepper to taste (optional)
1½ cups egg substitute
4 (6-inch) flour tortillas
Picante sauce (optional)
Fat-free sour cream (optional)

SERVES 4

3 GRAMS FAT
PER SERVING

Prep :10
Cook :20
Stand :00
Total :30

Brown the bacon in a large nonstick skillet until desired doneness. Turn out of the pan and blot any excess fat on a paper towel. Set aside.

Using the same skillet, wipe out any fat with a paper towel, and cook the potatoes until done, stirring often. Add salt and pepper to taste if desired. Return the bacon to the skillet and mix slightly with potatoes. Pour the egg substitute over the potatoes and bacon. After it begins to set, with a rubber spatula move it around a little to form large curds. Do not stir, or it will become too dry. Repeat this cooking procedure until done, or egg substitute is set and no longer runs. Remove from heat. Keep warm.

Warm the tortillas according to package directions and lay them on a work surface. Spoon some of the egg mixture evenly down the center of each tortilla, top with picante sauce, if desired, roll up, and serve immediately. A dollop of fat-free sour cream is also a nice touch.

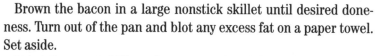

Variation: Chopped onions and bell peppers may be added to the potatoes to give a Western flair to the roll-ups. Use about ¼ cup each.

CAMPFIRE DELIGHT

This is not only for cooking over an open fire, but very good for an easy breakfast at home.

SERVES 4

4 GRAMS FAT
PER SERVING

Prep :05
Cook :15
Stand :03
Total :23

¾ cup diced low-fat ham (98% fat-free)
1 (16-ounce) package frozen potatoes, onions, and peppers, thawed
2 cups egg substitute
Salt and pepper (optional)
6 drops hot pepper sauce
¼ cup shredded fat-free Monterey Jack cheese
¼ cup shredded fat-free Cheddar cheese

Heat a nonstick skillet (if using a cast-iron skillet over an open fire, spray lightly with vegetable oil cooking spray). Add the ham and the potatoes with onions and peppers, cooking and stirring about 5 minutes. If they start to stick in the cast-iron pan, add a little water.

In a mixing bowl, combine the egg substitute, salt and pepper if desired, and hot pepper sauce. Pour into the skillet. Cover and cook for 8 to 10 minutes on medium-low heat or until set, lifting edges occasionally to let the uncooked part under as you would an omelet. Remove from heat, cover with cheeses, and let stand covered for 2 to 3 minutes, or until the cheeses are melted.

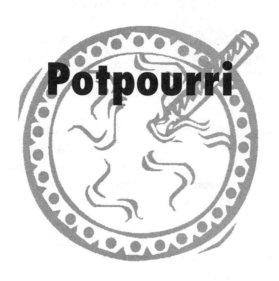

Potpourri

CHEESE SAUCE

SERVES 4

0 GRAMS FAT

Prep :10
Cook :06
Stand :00
Total :16

2 tablespoons nonfat dry milk powder
1 tablespoon all-purpose flour
¾ cup skim milk
4 slices fat-free American cheese, torn into pieces

In a saucepan, combine milk powder and flour; stir in the skim milk until smooth. Cook over medium heat until bubbly. Lower the heat to low and continue cooking and stirring about 1 minute more or until the sauce starts to thicken slightly. Stir in the cheese pieces, cooking until cheese melts

Serve over steamed veggies.

> *Variation:* White Sauce: Omit cheese and substitute ¼ cup butter-flavored sprinkles. Mix them with the dry milk and flour; continue recipe as directed.

CRANBERRY SAUCE

SERVES 4

0 GRAMS FAT

Prep :05
Cook :06
Stand :15
Total :26

1 (12-ounce) package fresh or frozen cranberries, thawed if frozen
½ cup plus 2 tablespoons sugar

Rinse fresh cranberries and pick over to remove bits of stem.

In a medium-size saucepan, combine sugar, cranberries, and 1 cup of water. Bring to a boil; continue cooking uncovered, stirring occasionally, for 5 to 6 minutes or until the berries pop and the mixture thickens slightly.

Transfer to a small serving bowl; cool slightly. Cover and refrigerate several hours or until cold.

HERB SAUCE

¾ cup plain nonfat yogurt
1 teaspoon honey
¾ teaspoon chopped fresh basil or ¼ teaspoon dried
¾ teaspoon chopped fresh tarragon leaves or ¼ teaspoon dried
¼ teaspoon salt
1 clove garlic, crushed
Pinch dried dill weed

SERVES 2

0 GRAMS FAT

Prep :05
Cook :00
Stand 2:00
Total 2:05

Mix all ingredients. Cover and refrigerate at least 2 hours but no longer than 24 hours.

Serve over steamed vegetables.

BAKED POTATO TOPPING

½ cup fat-free sour cream
½ cup plain nonfat yogurt
¼ cup chopped fresh scallions or chives
2 tablespoons chopped fresh parsley
1 tablespoon Dijon mustard
Salt and pepper to taste

SERVES 4

0 GRAMS FAT

Prep :05
Cook :00
Stand :00
Total :05

In a small bowl, combine all ingredients. Spoon some of the mixture over a split hot baked potato and serve.

Note: This makes about 1 cup, enough for 4, but at our house I make a double batch because we like lots of topping on our potatoes.

CHOCOLATE FUDGE

SERVES 8

**6 GRAMS FAT
ENTIRE RECIPE
IF NUTS
OMITTED**

**Prep :35
Cook :08
Stand :00
Total :43**

1½ cups sugar
½ cup skim milk
2 heaping tablespoons Hershey's unsweetened cocoa powder
¾ teaspoon vanilla extract
½ cup chopped walnuts or pecans

In a medium saucepan, mix the sugar and milk and bring to a boil over moderate heat, stirring constantly until sugar dissolves. Continue boiling *without stirring* until a candy thermometer reaches 236 degrees, or a drop of the mixture forms a soft ball in cold water.

Remove from the heat; add cocoa and vanilla. Beat only until the mixture reaches a pudding-like consistency. Stir in the nuts and pour onto a cookie sheet sprayed with vegetable oil cooking spray. Cool completely, cut into squares, and enjoy.

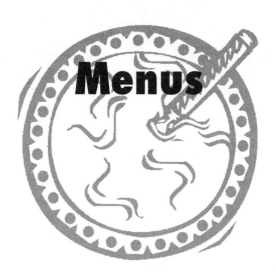

Menus

BREAKFAST I

0 GRAMS FAT

SERVES 1

This is for one person; you may adjust as needed. Just wanted you to see what a nice breakfast you can have with no fat.

	GRAMS FAT
Juice	0
Coffee (black)	0
Cereal with skim milk	0
Fresh fruit	0

BREAKFAST II

1 GRAM FAT

SERVES 1

	GRAMS FAT
Juice	0
Coffee (black)	0
Bagel	1
Cream cheese (fat-free)	0
Fresh fruit of choice	0

BREAKFAST III

1 GRAM FAT

SERVES 1

	GRAMS FAT
Juice	0
Coffee (black)	0
Maple French Toast	1 per serving
Fresh fruit cup	0

BRUNCH

7.75 GRAMS FAT PER SERVING

SERVES 8

	GRAMS FAT
Juice	0
Coffee (black)	0
Sausage and Grits for Breakfast	6.75 per serving
Scrambled egg substitute	0
Fruit of choice	0
Toast (dry) and jelly	1 per slice

CHRISTMAS MORNING

2 GRAMS FAT PER SERVING

SERVES 8

	GRAMS FAT
Champagne Orange Juice (double recipe)	0
Hot Chocolate Coffee (serves 1)	0
Christmas Morning French Toast	1 per serving
Hash Brown Breakfast Casserole	0
Coffee Cake	1 per serving

NEW YEAR'S BUFFET

4.67 GRAMS FAT PER SERVING

SERVES 8

*This is for 8 people; of course each recipe will
need adjusting to meet your specified needs,
according to the number of people
you are preparing for.*

	GRAMS FAT	SERVES
Country Caviar	0	12
Hot and Spicy Pepper Squares (people will eat more finger foods at a buffet—make plenty)	0	24
Mini Bagel Bits	0.5 per bagel	4 (double)
Quick Turkey Potpie	3 per serving	12
Tortilla Cheesecake	2 entire dish	12
Zippy Dip	0	8
Tater Dippers	0	6 (double)
Tortilla Chips	1 per serving	1 (8 times recipe)
Black-eyed peas	0	

PARTY BUFFET

6 GRAMS FAT PER SERVING

SERVES 8

	GRAMS FAT	SERVES
Mulled Cider	0	4 (double)
Pita Pizza Snacks	0	2 (4 times recipe)
White Bean Dip	0	4 (double)
Vegetable Dip	0	8

	GRAMS FAT	SERVES
Tortilla Chips	1 per serving	1 (8 times recipe)
Cranberry Salad	0	6 (double)
Sausage-Broccoli Casserole	1.5 per serving	8
Tasty Tomato Slices	1 per serving	6 (1½ times recipe)
Lemon Bread Pudding	2.5 per serving	4 (double)
Lemon Sauce	0	4 (double)

HOLIDAY ENTERTAINING

LESS THAN 14 GRAMS FAT PER SERVING

SERVES 8

	GRAMS FAT	SERVES
Christmas Wassail	0	10
Frozen Grapes	0	6 (1½ times recipe)
Vegetable Dip	0	8
Tortilla Chips	1 per serving	1 (8 times recipe)
Sweet Potato Chips	Trace of fat	4 (double)
Legal Eggnog	0	4 (double)
Frosty Wine Slush	0	4 (double)
Turkey, Rice, Sausage, and Cranberries All in One	Very low	8
Steamed broccoli and carrots	0	
Tasty Tomato Slices	1 per serving	6 (1½ times recipe)
Lemon Bread Pudding	2.5 per 1-cup serving	4 (double)
Lemon Sauce	0	4 (double)
Hot Chocolate Coffee	0	1 (8 times recipe)

MEXICAN DELIGHT

4.3 GRAMS FAT PER SERVING

SERVES 6

	GRAMS FAT	SERVES
Mexican Bean Pie	2.3 per serving	6
Tossed green salad with fat-free dressing	0	
Steamed whole-kernel corn	0	
Commercial baked tortilla chips, such as Frito Lay	1 per serving	
"I Worked All Day Making This Dessert"	1 per serving	Make according to number serving

CHILLY DAY COMPANY LUNCH

2.17 GRAMS FAT PER SERVING

SERVES 6

	GRAMS FAT	SERVES
Tossed green salad with fat-free dressing	0	
Broccoli Soup	0	6
Grilled Cheese Special	1.5 per serving	2 (triple)
Applicious Caramel Cake	0.67 per serving	12
Vanilla ice cream (fat-free)	0	

SUMMERTIME DINING

3 GRAMS FAT PER SERVING

SERVES 4

This is a cool delightful evening for guests as well as the hostess.

	GRAMS FAT	SERVES
Chicken Waldorf Salad	3 per serving	4
Fresh tomato slices	0	
Fresh fruit compote	0	

> *Tip:* For a summertime dessert, serve a fruit compote using in-season melons and serve in a watermelon bowl. Cut the watermelon in half the long way, hollow out one of the halves, and cut around the edge in a zigzag pattern (like sawteeth). Fill with balls made out of all different melons: cantaloupe, muskmelon, watermelon, etc. You can even use yellow and red watermelon, which is very pretty.

SUNDAY DELIGHT

5 GRAMS FAT PER SERVING

SERVES 4

Put the chicken in the oven on low before leaving for church. Make the salad before you leave; make the broccoli and rice when you return. Lunch is served! (Make the cake a day ahead. If there is any left, serve for lunch.)

	GRAMS FAT	SERVES
Tossed green salad with fat-free dressing	0	
Sweet and Tart Chicken	2.5 per serving	4
Quick Broccoli and Rice	1 per serving	2 (double)
Bread of your choice (be careful of fat grams— choose wisely)		
Strawberry Sundae Cake	1.5 per serving	12

FAMILY DINNER

2 GRAMS FAT PER SERVING

SERVES 4

This is an "I'm really tired, get me out of the kitchen" dinner.

	GRAMS FAT	SERVES
Grilled Chicken Cheese Sandwich	2 per serving	4
Corn and Broccoli	0	4
Fat-free ice cream or yogurt	0	

> *Tip:* Most of my recipes are quick and easy, as I do *not* have time to spare, but I still want good food and to look good when I entertain my friends. Most of my friends appreciate the fact that they are eating healthy at my house, and so will yours.

DINNER MENU

A TAD LESS THAN 5 GRAMS FAT PER SERVING

SERVES 4

	GRAMS FAT	SERVES
Tossed green salad with fat-free dressing	0	
Chicken Vegetable Special	4 per serving	4
Mexican Corn Bread	0.05 per serving	8
Amaretto Rice Pudding	<1 per serving	6

CAJUN CASUAL

LESS THAN 7 GRAMS FAT PER SERVING

SERVES 8

	GRAMS FAT	SERVES
Relish tray: veggie sticks, pickles, peppers, etc.	0	
Bayou Magic Chicken	3 per serving	8
Short-cut Beans and Rice	<1 per serving	4 (double)
Chips or bread of your choice (read the label and count your grams)		
Chocolate Bread Pudding	2.5 per serving	4 (double)
Chocolate Sauce	Trace of fat	2 (4 times recipe)

DINNER MENU

6.29 GRAMS FAT PER SERVING

SERVES 4

	GRAMS FAT	SERVES
Tossed green salad with fat-free dressing	0	
Miracle Chicken	3 per serving	4
Corn and Potato Casserole	4.75 entire dish	6
Bread of your choice		
Lemon Bread Pudding	2.5 per serving	4
Lemon Sauce	0	4

DINNER IN ONE

	GRAMS FAT	SERVES
Bean Burrito Casserole (this includes salad and vegetables; see recipe)	<4 per serving	4
Scoop of fat-free ice cream topped with a little Kahlúa	0	

Hints and Tips

1. Keep a jar of whole nutmegs and a small grater on your spice shelf. Just a sprinkle or two will perk up the flavor on steamed vegetables, mashed potatoes, and rice, for example.
2. Try "cutting" experimenting while in the kitchen. When baking, *cut* back on the amount of butter, margarine, and shortening, or *cut* them out. Often, low-fat yogurt or buttermilk can substitute for the missing fats without noticeable difference. (How do you think we write cookbooks? Everything we eat is an experiment and sometimes an experience.)
3. Marinate your boneless skinless chicken breast in fruit juices flavored with light low-sodium soy sauce, flavored with spices or herbs instead of the oil-based marinades. Try: orange juice with tarragon, pineapple juice with rosemary, or apple juice with ground or fresh ginger.
4. The next time you bake a cake from a mix, try substituting an equal amount of applesauce for the shortening called for on the package and an equal amount of egg substitute for the number of eggs called for (¼ cup = 1 egg). You'll trim a good-sized amount of fat grams just by doing this. Don't tell—no one will know the difference.
5. Try using balsamic vinegar, which has almost no trace at all of fat or calories, sprinkled on a baked potato. More restaurants will probably have this than fat-free dressing, although some are starting to carry fat-free dressing as well as many other items. *Ask* every time you eat out. The more we ask, the more they will help us out. Balsamic vinegar, used sparingly, will also add a special touch to your salad dressings, marinades, pastas, and meats. The best has a sweet-tart, oak-aged blend of flavors and a syrupy consistency.
6. Keep a shaker of confectioners' sugar mixed with ground cinnamon and cloves handy. Use it instead of butter or margarine to dust pancakes, waffles, oatmeal, acorn squash, steamed squash, toast. Again, I say, experiment!

7. Grate the zest (peel) of your citrus fruits after squeezing; store in a zipper-lock plastic bag and freeze to spark up fish, chicken, salads, vegetables, and desserts.

8. Try out some of the prepared mustards. Many are fat-free and will spice up everything from salad dressing to dips.

9. Shake butter-flavored granules over hot moist foods to get the butter flavor that so many of us desire. There are many flavors to choose from—garlic, sour cream, cheese, regular, and no telling what by the time this book gets published. The market has something new every day. I found fat-free wieners yesterday.

10. Use crunchy nugget-type cereals as stand-ins for nuts in batters and for toppings also.

11. If you want to thicken your gravy, sauces, and soups, try puréed vegetables instead of fat and flour; use potatoes, dried peas, winter squash, beans, etc. If you are making a stew, just take some of the vegetables out, place in the blender, purée, and return to the stew to thicken the remaining liquid.

12. Think you are going to die without whipped cream during the holidays? Try whipping evaporated skim milk, and add a touch of vanilla extract or confectioners' sugar for added richness. The secret is get the milk, bowl, and beaters very cold before starting to whip, and it will whip just like cream. Remember, don't tell.

13. Try a little jelly or marmalade thinned with fruit juice as a glaze for meat. Hot pepper jelly is also a nice spicy touch.

14. Use commercial fat-free salad dressings for more than just your salad. Try them on your baked potato, on steamed vegetables, or as a dip. They are great and quick for parties. You may even decide to experiment and add a little more fat-free mayonnaise or Miracle Whip, a little balsamic vinegar, a spicy mustard—or just use them straight out of the bottle.

15. As you will notice after reading some of the recipes in this and in my first book, my nonstick skillet is indispensable. *Break* the fry habit but keep out the skillet; you can do wonders with a nonstick pan. Without the stick of butter, you can do wonders getting into last year's jeans.

16. If you hate vegetables like my friend Shirley, you can get your daily dose in a concealed way. (This is also good for fooling kids into getting their needed amount of veggies.) Dice or shred zucchini, carrots, bell peppers, eggplant, onions, mushrooms, or just about any vegetable and add to your spaghetti sauce. This is one thing almost all kids will eat and so will Shirley. What she doesn't know won't hurt her. (Ha ha, Shirley. Be careful what you think you're eating at my house.)

17. Keep a roll of heavy aluminum foil handy in the summer. Place a few vegetables of your choice, such as onion, carrots, peppers, whatever is in season, on top of a chicken cutlet or chicken tender or a piece of fish. Sprinkle some wine over all, or some fat-free chicken broth. (Remember I told you in my first book to keep a can in your pantry for quick fixings.) Fold and crimp the foil edges to form a packet, place on the grill, and cook your entire meal in one. You can also do this on a cookie sheet in a hot oven, about 400 degrees.

18. Keep a bag of sun-dried tomatoes on hand. Choose the ones you simply soak in water instead of the ones packed in oil. Cut them into slivers or dice fine and add to pasta dishes, chicken, and vegetable dishes. They will also add a very nice flavor to pasta salads. Remember where I live—Gore, America—so I can only get these when I go to town. That is what we say down here in the South when we go into the city. But I do have fun going to the grocery stores in the city, as much fun as to the clothing department stores (I lied), oops!

19. Fresh herbs make a world of difference in the taste of your dish. You can plant small pots of basil, oregano, sage, rosemary, parsley, and other fragrant varieties and keep them on your kitchen windowsill. You get much enjoyment out of having your own home-grown herbs. I guess being a farmer's daughter shows I do like to grow things myself (although it's much easier to filch off brother).

20. If you desire bacon crumbles on salads or on your sandwich, cook turkey bacon crisp, crumble it, and use instead of regular bacon. Much less fat, same flavor.

21. Eat beans at least twice a week. They are great heart food, are rich in protein and fiber but lean in fat. Red meat, on the other hand, is one of the highest sources of fat and contains no fiber. It is fine to eat meat in moderation—that's your choice—but you can fill up on

beans (legumes) such as white, pinto, (brown) navy, chick-peas, lentils, butter, lima, whatever kind you choose. This brings me to another story.

My escort in one of the cities I toured in with Simon & Schuster last year had never heard of eating a bowl of beans. This young lady is in for a real surprise. She asked me if it took a while to acquire a taste for them and how could anyone sit down and eat a whole bowl of just beans. I couldn't believe my ears. Poor girl, I just think of how much gas she has missed out on during her lifetime. Why, I can't imagine. I felt so sorry for her, I just think I will Fed-Ex her a quart of good home-cooked brown beans. She may move to Oklahoma, or the involuntary gastric explosion may move her out here before she is quite ready. Bless her heart, I love her anyway, even if she doesn't know "beans."

22. Eat a carrot and an orange every day. Researchers are convinced that eating foods high in antioxidant nutrients—including vitamins C and E and beta-carotene—may help prevent heart disease, cancer, and other chronic diseases associated with aging. (I think I will eat two a day.) Carrots are loaded with beta-carotene, oranges with vitamin C. Other foods rich in antioxidants are broccoli, cantaloupe, apricots, spinach, sweet potatoes, and winter squash.

23. You know I hate three things: fruit, fish, and exercise. Even so, I am encouraging you to do all three. Do as I say, not as I do. You should also try to eat fresh fruit instead of just drinking the fruit juice. Juice is a breakfast favorite, but if you eat the whole fruit not only do you get a fiber boost when choosing fruit over juice but eating a piece of fruit takes longer to consume—which tricks you into feeling as if you've eaten more. I will eat an orange, a grapefruit, or an apple on occasion but the other fruits I can't handle. Then again, do as I say. (I do make myself drink orange juice in the morning, so I do practice what I preach. Just had you fooled, didn't I?)

24. Try to include pasta in your diet at least three times a week. It is low in fat as well as filling. Try a cold pasta salad for lunch. Pasta contains any needed B-complex vitamins, iron, and calcium. It is cholesterol-free with the exception of egg noodles—stay away from those—remember eggs are a no-no. Pasta contains little sodium. Use skim milk

instead of cream when making white sauces for pasta; use cheese sparingly as a flavor accent, and make it a low-fat or fat-free cheese. Look for prepared tomato sauce that is made without oil, such as Healthy Choice. If you count calories, a serving of 2 ounces of pasta will contain only 210 calories. I don't count calories, but if you care to do this it is fine. There again, let me say you have to make up *your* mind what you are going to do and then the rest is easy. *Making up your mind* is the key to success in anything you do. If you don't, you are wasting your time.

25. Butter Buds: I use lots of liquid-form Butter Buds in my recipes, and I guess that the most asked question I have heard is "What are liquid-form Butter Buds and where do you get them?" These are granules or sprinkles, and are in a shaker-top container, but they also are in box mix form, and can be used either way. They are in envelopes that have instructions on how much water to add to each. A number you can call if you cannot find them or have questions is (800) 231-1123, or in New York State, (800) 336-0363.

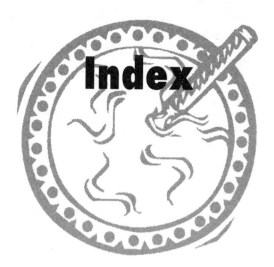

Index